7-2-24

Baillière's

CLINICAL OBSTETRICS AND GYNAECOLOGY

INTERNATIONAL PRACTICE AND RESEARCH

Baillière's

CLINICAL
OBSTETRICS
AND
GYNAECOLOGY

INTERNATIONAL PRACTICE AND RESEARCH

Volume 10/Number 3
September 1996

The Menopause: Key Issues

D. H. BARLOW MA, BSc, MD, FRCOG
Guest Editor

Baillière Tindall
London Philadelphia Sydney Tokyo Toronto

This book is printed on acid-free paper.

Baillière Tindall 24–28 Oval Road
W.B. Saunders London NW1 7DX, UK
Company Ltd
The Curtis Center, Independence Square West,
Philadelphia, PA 19106–3399, USA

55 Horner Avenue
Toronto, Ontario M8Z 4X6, Canada

Harcourt Brace & Company
Australia
30–52 Smidmore Street, Marrickville, NSW 2204, Australia

Harcourt Brace & Company
Japan Inc
Ichibancho Central Building,
22–1 Ichibancho, Chiyoda-ku, Tokyo 102, Japan

Whilst great care has been taken to maintain the accuracy of the information contained in this issue, the authors, editor, owners and publishers cannot accept any responsibility for any loss or damage arising from actions or decisions based on information contained in this publication; ultimate responsibility for the treatment of patients and interpretation of published material lies with the medical practitioner. The opinions expressed are those of the authors and the inclusion in this publication of material relating to a particular product, method or technique does not amount to an endorsement of its value or quality, or of the claims made by its manufacturer.

ISSN 0950–3552

ISBN 0–7020–2177–6 (single copy)

Baillière's Clinical Obstetrics and Gynaecology is published four times each year by Baillière Tindall. Prices for Volume 10 (1996) are:

TERRITORY	ANNUAL SUBSCRIPTION	SINGLE ISSUE
Europe including UK	£102.00 (Institutional) post free	£30.00 post free
	£87.00 (Individual) post free	
All other countries	Consult your local Harcourt Brace & Company office	

The editor of this publication is Gail Greensmith, Baillière Tindall, 24–28 Oval Road, London NW1 7DX, UK.

Baillière's Clinical Obstetrics and Gynaecology is covered in Index Medicus, Current Contents/ Clinical Medicine, the Science Citation Index, SciSearch, Research Alert and Excerpta Medica.

Baillière's Clinical Obstetrics and Gynaecology was published from 1983 to 1986 as *Clinics in Obstetrics and Gynaecology*

Typeset by Phoenix Photosetting, Chatham.
Printed and bound in Great Britain by the University Printing House, Cambridge, UK.

Contributors to this issue

DAVID H. BARLOW MA, BSc, MD, FRCOG, Nuffield Professor of Obstetrics and Gynaecology, University of Oxford, John Radcliffe Hospital, Headley Way, Headington, Oxford OX3 9DU, UK.

CAROLYN M. BEALE BSc, Clinical Physiologist, Imperial College School of Medicine at the National, Heart & Lung Institute, and Royal Brompton Hospital, Dovehouse Street, London SW3 6LY, UK.

HENRY G. BURGER AO, MD, BS, FRACP, FCP(SA), FRACOG, FRCP(UK), FAA, Director, Prince Henry's Institute of Medical Research, PO Box 5152, Clayton, Victoria 3168, Australia.

PETER COLLINS MA, MD, FRCP, FESC, FACC, Senior Lecturer and Honorary Consultant Cardiologist, Imperial College School of Medicine at the National, Heart & Lung Institute, and Royal Brompton Hospital, Dovehouse Street, London SW3 6LY, UK.

J. ANDREW FANTL MD, Professor and Vice Chairman, Department of Obstetrics, Gynecology & Reproductive Medicine, University Medical Center at Stony Brook, HSC T-9, Room 033, Stony Brook, NY 11794, USA.

KEITH HAWTON DM, FRCPsych, Professor of Psychiatry, Consultant, University Department of Psychiatry, Warneford Hospital, Oxford OX3 7JX, UK.

JOHN A. KANIS MD, FRCP, FRCPath, Professor in Human Metabolism & Clinical Biochemistry, University of Sheffield; Honorary Consultant Physician, Royal Hallamshire Hospital, Medical School, Beech Hill Road, Sheffield S10 2RX, UK.

MARY-JANE PEARCE BMedSci, BMBS, MRCGP, MRCPsych, Consultant Psychiatrist, Littlemore Hospital, Littlemore, Oxon OX4 4XN, UK.

MARGARET C. P. REES MA, DPhil, MRCOG, Honorary Senior Clinical Lecturer in Obstetrics and Gynaecology, John Radcliffe Hospital, Women's Centre, Headington, Oxford OX3 9DU, UK.

JOSEPH SCHAFFER MD, Assistant Professor, Department of Obstetrics, Gynecology & Reproductive Medicine, University Medical Center at Stony Brook, HSC T-9, Room 033, Stony Brook, NY 11794, USA.

JOHN C. STEVENSON MBBS, FRCP, Senior Lecturer and Honorary Consultant Physician, Wynn Division of Metabolic Research, Imperial College School of Medicine at the National Heart and Lung Institute, Cecil Rosen Research Laboratories, 21 Wellington Road, London NW8 9SQ, UK.

MALCOLM WHITEHEAD MBBS, FRCOG, Consultant Gynaecologist, Menopause Clinic, Kings College School of Medicine & Dentistry, London SE5 9RX, UK.

BARRY G. WREN MD, BS, MHPEd, FRACOG, FRCOG, Director, Centre for Management of the Menopause, Royal Hospital for Women, Paddington, Sydney; Professor, Eastpoint Tower, Suite 506, 180 Ocean Street, Edge Cliff, NSW 2027, Australia.

Table of contents

PREVIOUS ISSUES

FORTHCOMING ISSUE

Preface

There was a time when the field of the menopause and hormone replacement therapy was very much a minority interest within gynaecology but that is no longer the case. Interest generated by the increasing diversity of therapeutic options and the explosion of information on the positive and negative effects of HRT have helped raise the profile of this field substantially, both within the health care professions, with the general public, with the media, and with the pharmaceutical industry. Along with this interest there have been a number of volumes reviewing the field, particularly with emphasis on hormone replacement therapy.

Rather than focus on hormone replacement therapy this issue concentrates on the biology of menopause and its consequences although it is inevitable that this will include up-to-date information on hormone replacement therapy. I have brought together a group of authors who are expert in their fields and who have provided authoritative reviews on important aspects of the menopause. The range of the subjects covered emphasizes the diverse expertise involved in the health care of the menopausal woman. This is now a multidisciplinary field but it is essential that gynaecologists retain an awareness of the whole field since we are frequently asked to provide women with advice across that whole field. This issue provides an important update.

D. H. BARLOW

1

The menopausal transition

HENRY G. BURGER

During the past decade or more, attention has focused on the menopause and the consequences of oestrogen deprivation, particularly on cardio-vascular and bony health, and lately on brain function and the occurrence of dementia. Currently, increasing efforts are being made to improve our understanding of the years just prior to the menopause. The menopause is defined by the World Health Organization as the permanent cessation of menstruation resulting from the loss of ovarian follicular activity. The term perimenopause is used to describe that period beginning with the first symptoms or indications of the approaching menopause and ending 12 months after the final menstrual period. The term 'menopausal transition' describes that part of the perimenopause ending at the final menstrual period. A prospective study of 2570 North American women, aged 44 to 55, followed for five years by McKinlay et al (1992), showed that menstrual irregularity commenced on average at 47.5 years of age and the duration of the transition was almost four years. In this chapter, a review of the key elements of the pituitary–ovarian axis is followed by a discussion of the size of the ovarian follicle pool and its changes with ageing, and a description of the endocrine changes which have been reported during the menopausal transition. Symptoms associated with the transition and the consequences of changing hormone levels are reviewed briefly.

THE PITUITARY–OVARIAN AXIS

In a simplified summary of current concepts, ovarian function, comprising oocyte development and hormone production, is under the dual control of the pituitary gonadotropins, follicle stimulating hormone (FSH) and luteinizing hormone (LH). LH is under the major control of hypothalamic gonadotropin releasing hormone (GnRH), is secreted in a pulsatile manner, and is under the negative feedback control of oestradiol and progesterone for much of the cycle, whilst a positive feedback mechanism operates to generate the mid-cycle LH surge which triggers ovulation. The study of LH has not contributed a great deal to our current understanding of the menopausal transition and LH will not be dealt with further. FSH is also

Baillière's Clinical Obstetrics and Gynaecology—
Vol. 10, No. 3, September 1996
ISBN 0–7020–2177–6
0950–3552/96/030347 + 13 $12.00/00

347

under the partial control of GnRH, but has an important component of autonomous secretion, independent of GnRH, and involving the local action of activin (see below). FSH is under dual ovarian negative feedback control by the gonadal peptide inhibin as well as by the steroid hormones, in particular oestradiol, and progesterone.

The major source of circulating oestradiol during a normal menstrual cycle is the dominant follicle, although its intercycle levels are maintained by the cohort of growing follicles.

Inhibin is the generic name given to a family of gonadal glycoprotein hormones with a dimeric structure (Burger, 1992). Two major inhibin species, A and B, are found in man, consisting of a common α-subunit and one of two different β-subunits, $β_A$ and $β_B$. The major biological function of the inhibins is to suppress the synthesis and/or secretion of FSH by direct pituitary action. The activins, however, are dimers of the β-subunits and, as opposed to the major long loop feedback endocrine action of the inhibins, are probably more important in paracrine and autocrine activities. Paradoxically, activins have the property of stimulating rather than inhibiting FSH, and a local intrapituitary mechanism, involving activin, underlies the autonomous component of FSH secretion. The biological activities of activin are modulated by a third gonadal peptide, follistatin, which has activin binding properties.

Both inhibin and oestradiol are products of ovarian granulosa cells. Whereas the dominant follicle is a major source of circulating oestradiol, studies of ovarian venous inhibin concentrations have shown that the ovarian vein:peripheral vein gradient is similar on the side of the dominant follicle and on the contralateral side, indicating that ovarian follicles other than the dominant follicle contribute importantly to circulating inhibin concentrations (lllingworth et al, 1991). This observation is the basis for the hypothesis of differential regulation of FSH by inhibin and oestradiol, considered in further detail below.

The majority of observations regarding inhibin physiology have been based on a radioimmunoassay widely referred to as the 'Monash assay' (Burger, 1993). This assay is known to cross-react with non-biologically active α-subunit precursors as well as with biologically active A and B inhibins. The levels of inhibin immunoreactivity measured using this assay, fluctuate during the menstrual cycle. They are relatively constant throughout most of the follicular phase, with a small mid-cycle surge and a subsequent and larger luteal phase peak which is parallel to the rise and fall of luteal progesterone and oestradiol (McLachlan et al, 1987). Measurements using an assay specific for inhibin A have shown a pattern of secretion qualitatively similar to that using the Monash assay (Groome et al, 1994). Very recently, an inhibin B assay has been developed and preliminary reports suggest that the pattern of inhibin B secretion differs from that of inhibin A, with an intercycle rise and subsequent fall late in the follicular phase, with low levels throughout the luteal phase. Descriptions of inhibin physiology during the menopausal transition are based on the Monash assay, with no data currently available regarding the behaviour of inhibin B at that time.

AGEING AND THE SIZE OF THE OVARIAN FOLLICLE POOL

The number of primordial follicles in the human ovary is maximal during fetal life. After birth, there is a steady decline in follicle numbers with increasing age, until approximately 38 years. The rate of decline then increases markedly and by the time of the final menstrual period, follicles are virtually absent from the ovaries. The relationship of follicle numbers to the occurrence of the menopausal transition and the menopause was clarified by Richardson et al (1987). They studied 17 women, aged 44 to 55 years, divided on the basis of whether they were still cycling regularly, were in the menopausal transition or were post-menopausal. The ovaries of regularly cycling subjects contained, on average, about 1000 primordial follicles, those in the transition approximately 100 follicles, whilst in four post-menopausal women only one follicle was identified in one of eight ovaries examined. Thus a very marked decline in follicle numbers provides the morphological basis for changes occurring during the menopausal transition (Figure 1).

The precise mechanisms involved in the decline in follicle numbers and the marked increase in the rate of follicle loss around 38 years of age are uncertain. Faddy and Gosden (1995) developed a mathematical model to describe the rates of growth and death of follicles in women aged 19 to 50 years. The accelerated decline in follicle numbers was postulated to result from an increase in the rate of atresia of primordial follicles. Their model predicted that the number of follicles growing from a stage at which there are at least two layers of granulosa cells surrounding an oocyte, decreases from 51 per day at 24 to 25 years of age to only one per day at 49 to 50 years of age. We can hypothesize that the decline in follicle growth and development might be reflected in declining levels of inhibin production by such follicles.

Studies of the hormonal changes which occur with age in regularly cycling women suggest that there is a progressive increase in FSH levels from 29 to 30 years of age onwards (Ahmed Ebbiary et al, 1994). Several other groups have documented the increase in serum FSH levels with increasing age, the most extensive study being that of Lee et al (1988) who investigated 94 regularly cycling women aged 24 to 50 years. They showed that FSH levels during the follicular phase and early post-ovulatory period rose significantly with increasing age, despite the lack of any significant change in LH until close to the age of 50 years. Their study showed no significant change in the levels of circulating oestradiol. The increasing FSH levels which have been reported appear to be inverse to the declining follicle numbers. If it is accepted that no significant change in oestradiol levels occurs during this period, it can be hypothesized that serum inhibin levels might also fall in proportion to declining follicle numbers and might thus allow FSH levels to rise. Such rising FSH levels might in turn provide the additional drive for the maintenance of circulating oestradiol. Some experimental support for a change in immunoreactive inhibin with increasing age has been provided by MacNaughton et al (1992). They

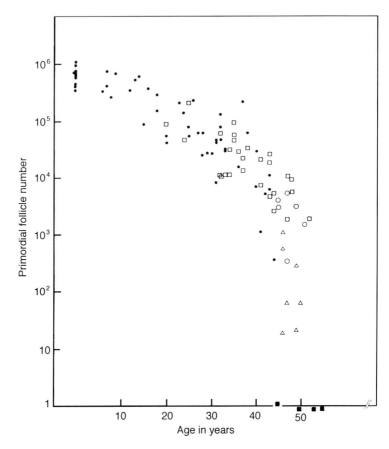

Figure 1. Relationship between age and primordial follicle number compared using data from ●, Block (1952, 1953); □, Gougeon (1984) and Richardson et al (1987). ○, regular; △, perimenopausal; ■, post-menopausal. Reproduced from Richardson et al (1987, *Journal of Clinical Endocrinology and Metabolism* **65:** 1231–1237 © The Endocrine Society) with permission.

studied follicular phase levels of gonadotropins and oestradiol in normal volunteers sampled on a single occasion during the follicular phase of the cycle and showed that inhibin fell as age increased (Figure 2).

Following complete follicle depletion, which occurs at the final menstrual period, it would be predicted that circulating oestradiol and inhibin concentrations would be very low, allowing a marked rise in circulating FSH. This is of course the endocrine picture characteristic of the post-menopausal state, with FSH levels being 10 to 15 times higher than follicular phase levels during reproductive life, oestradiol levels being 10% or less of reproductive age concentration and inhibin being, in general, undetectable.

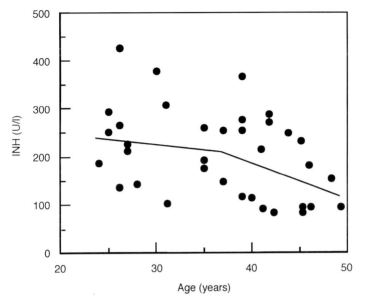

Figure 2. Change in inhibin (INH) levels with age in women in the follicular phase of the menstrual cycle. The continuous line represents the robust locally-weighted regression (LOWESS). Reproduced from MacNaughton et al (1992, *Clinical Endocrinology* **36**: 339–345, Blackwell Science Ltd.) with permission.

HORMONAL CHANGES DURING THE MENOPAUSAL TRANSITION

The menopausal transition is a time when menstrual cycles become highly variable both in regularity and flow (Sherman et al, 1979). Whilst the median length of the menstrual cycle falls from 30 days at 25 years of age to 28 days at 35 years of age, resulting primarily from a shortening of the follicular phase, the immediate post-menarchial phase as well as the pre-menopausal phase are times of marked variability in cycle length. When basal body temperature has been used to detect the presence of ovulation, it is clear that anovulatory cycles become more prevalent with the approach of the menopause, for example 3 to 7% of cycles were reported as anovulatory between the ages of 26 and 40 years and 12 to 15% between the ages of 41 and 50 years (Doring, 1969). When luteal phase progesterone levels are measured, the frequency of non-detectable concentrations increases gradually as the final menstrual period approaches. In a large study of peri-menopausal hormone levels (Rannevik et al, 1995), the frequency of cycles with progesterone levels indicative of ovulation (concentrations >10 nmol/l) decreased from 60% to less than 10% during the six years preceding the final menstrual period. Ovulatory progesterone levels were observed in 62% of women 72 to 61 months prior to the final menstrual period, but in only 4.8% of those within six to nine months of the menopause, whilst all progesterone levels were <2 nmol/l post-menopausally.

There is in fact only a small amount of hormonal data available, focusing specifically on the menopausal transition. Sherman and Korenman (1975) recorded hormone levels daily in two women, one aged 49 and the other 50 who were in the menopausal transition. Two of the cycles were anovulatory, but were characterized by gradually increasing levels of oestradiol and initially post-menopausal levels of FSH and LH, which fell subsequently as oestradiol rose. The anovulatory cycle described in one of these subjects was followed by a cycle that demonstrated evidence of follicular maturation. Additional studies were repeated by the same investigators (Sherman et al, 1979).

Metcalf et al (1981) examined the concentrations of FSH, LH, oestrogen and pregnandiol in weekly urine samples collected from 14 to 87 weeks, from 31 perimenopausal women aged 36 to 55. They emphasized the marked variability of these levels. Hee et al (1993) reported gonadotropin, oestradiol and immunoreactive inhibin concentrations in a longitudinal study of three volunteers early in their menopausal transition, at 45 and 46 years of age. They described abrupt declines in oestradiol and inhibin into the post-menopausal range, with inverse changes in FSH and LH, with subsequent levels characteristic of women of reproductive age. Again, hormonal variability was the major aspect emphasized by this study (Figure 3). A recent publication has provided further descriptions of the hormonal changes during the transition, in relation to self-reported menstrual cycle status (Burger et al, 1995). In this study, termed the Melbourne Mid-life Project, a population sample of 437 women was recruited following a cross-sectional survey of a randomly selected group of 2001 Australian born Melbourne women, aged between 45 and 55 and initially interviewed in May 1991 (Dennerstein et al, 1993). Blood samples were obtained between the fourth and eighth day of the menstrual cycle, for measurements of FSH, oestradiol and immunoreactive inhibin. The data obtained in the first year of this current longitudinal study were subjected to cross-sectional analysis. Twenty-seven per cent of the subjects had reported no change in menstrual frequency or flow and were taken as the control group, relative to whom changes in the remaining groups were analysed. Twenty-three per cent had reported a change in menstrual flow without change in frequency, 9% a change in frequency without any change in flow and 28% a change both in frequency and flow. In 13%, no menses had been reported for at least three months. FSH levels were lowest in the control group and progressively increased in the other four groups, being most marked in those experiencing changes in frequency and flow and in those that had not bled for three months or more. Oestradiol levels were lower in the groups experiencing a change in frequency or frequency and flow, but were statistically significantly lower only in those who had not had a bleed for at least three months. In that group the geometric mean oestradiol concentration was 42% of that in the control group (Figure 4). It is noteworthy that there was a wide range in oestradiol concentrations. Immunoreactive inhibin levels were also reduced in those experiencing a change in frequency and flow and were 38% of those in the control group with three or more months of amenorrhoea. Analysis of the hormone levels in terms of age showed progressive rises in FSH (11.8% per year) and falls in oestradiol and inhibin (7.8% and 9.9% per year, respectively). From a practical view point, it is important to note that 43% of the subjects who reported no change in menstrual cycle characteristics had FSH levels higher than those of young normal subjects at the same stage of the follicular phase of the cycle, whilst 94% of those who had not bled for three months or more had elevated FSH levels. Even more importantly, 6% of those

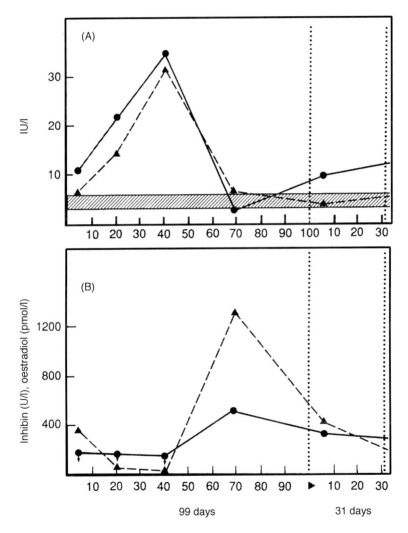

Figure 3. A, ●—●, follicle stimulating hormone; ▲—▲, luteinizing hormone. B, ●—●, inhibin (U/l); and ▲—▲ oestradiol (pmol/l) levels in a 45-year-old normal volunteer studied in the first cycle of her menopausal transition. Hormone levels typical of post-menopausal values are followed by levels occurring during reproductive life. Reproduced from Hee et al (1993, *Maturitas* **18**: 9–20) with permission.

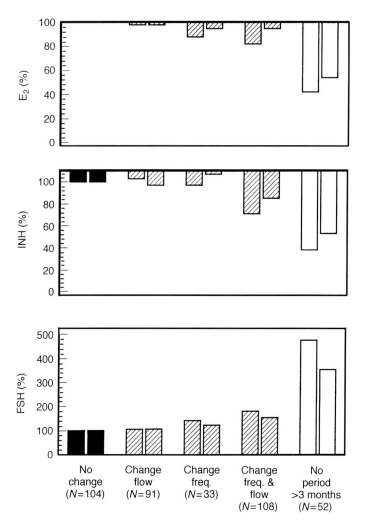

Figure 4. Changes in oestradiol (E_2); inhibin (INH); and follicle stimulating hormone (FSH), as a percentage of levels in group 1 women from the Melbourne Mid-Life Project who had experienced no change in their menstrual cycles. The left column is unadjusted and the right is adjusted for age and body mass index. Adapted from the data of Burger et al (1995, *Journal of Clinical Endocrinology and Metabolism* **80**: 3537–3545, © The Endocrine Society) with permission.

without any change in menstrual cycle status had FSH levels in the range typically found post-menopausally, as did 33% of those with a change in menstrual cycle frequency and 76% of those who had not bled for three months. Twenty-four per cent of women in the control group had oestradiol levels lower than those normally found in the follicular phase in young women, rising to 60% of those who had not bled for three months, whilst inhibin levels were low in 22% of the control group and 81% of the group who had three or more months of amenorrhoea. A hyperbolic relationship was noted between FSH and both oestradiol and inhibin, both of which were significantly inversely correlated with FSH.

In considering the hormonal changes associated with the menopausal transition, it is important to note the few published investigations of gonadotropin and steroid levels considered relative to the final menstrual period. Rannevik et al (1995) reported data from 160 women in the Malmö perimenopausal project (Figure 5). They had been sampled regularly over a period of 12 years centred on the final menses. Again a continuous increase in serum FSH and LH was noted from 4.75 years prior to the final menstrual period, the increase continuing to at least the first sample after that point, the sampling interval being six months. Oestradiol was measured for seven years prior to the final menstrual period and remained relatively constant (mean levels between 461 and 515 pmol/l) until the sample obtained six months prior to the final menses. In 154 observations one to six months before that last period, oestradiol was still found to average 383 pmol/l but had fallen by more than 50% in the one to six months after the final menses with a further gradual fall to 171 pmol/l at seven to 12 months. By 97 to 108 months later, oestradiol levels were much lower, at 72 pmol/l. The data thus confirm other studies which show a 10- to 15-fold increase in serum FSH after the final menses, a three- to fivefold increase in LH and a more than 80% drop in oestradiol during that time. Rannevik et al (1995) did not characterize their subjects according to menstrual cycle status, but did report on the increased frequency of inadequate luteal function during the immediately pre-menopausal period.

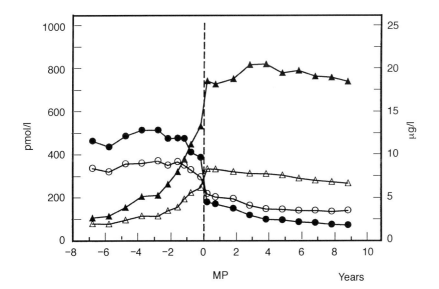

Figure 5. Mean serum levels of ▲, follicle stimulating hormone; △, luteinizing hormone; ●, oestradiol; ⊖, oestrone during the perimenopausal transition. Reproduced from Rannevik et al (1995, *Maturitas* **21:** 103–113) with permission.

Overall it can be stated that the menopausal transition is a time of markedly fluctuating hormone levels when individual subjects are followed. Cross-sectional data on groups of women, however, show relative preservation of oestradiol and inhibin concentrations until close to the final menstrual period when data from single time point analyses are considered. The most striking and characteristic endocrine feature of the menopausal transition is the progressive and fluctuating increase in serum FSH. This is most plausibly explained on the basis of decreased ovarian feedback and it may well be that during the menopausal transition, integrated levels of oestradiol and inhibin are falling inversely to the rise in FSH. The fluctuating and presumably falling hormone levels are likely to be the underlying cause of the symptoms as well as other changes observed during the menopausal transition (fall in bone mineral density, changes in serum lipids).

SYMPTOMS ASSOCIATED WITH THE MENOPAUSAL TRANSITION

Whilst there is a wide variation in the frequency with which women from different ethnic groups and different socioeconomic and educational backgrounds report the occurrence of symptoms associated with the menopause, most studies show that there is an increase in symptom reporting during the menopausal transition. These include the classic vasomotor symptoms of hot flushes, with or without night sweats, a variety of psychological and psychosomatic complaints not so clearly tied to menopausal status, and disturbances of sexuality. In those populations where symptom reporting is prevalent (e.g. Australia, Canada and the USA), there is a marked increase in symptoms during the perimenopause (Dennerstein et al, 1993). In addition to classic symptoms, some women report features suggestive of high oestrogen levels, such as bloating and breast tenderness. These may reflect the marked fluctuations in perimenopausal oestrogens with levels occasionally rising well above 1000 to 1500 pmol/l. The occurrence of such symptoms and their underlying pathophysiology suggests that hormonal supplementation at this time is likely to be effective. A logical and plausible approach is the use of low-dose combined oral contraceptive pills, which would be expected to suppress gonadotropin secretion and markedly decrease the hormonal fluctuations.

It is noteworthy that several cross-sectional European studies have reported that a sense of wellbeing was lowest and negative psychological symptoms highest among women in the perimenopausal period relative to those judged pre- or post-menopausal (e.g. Hunter et al, 1986). A recent North American longitudinal study of women going through the menopausal transition (Matthews et al, 1994) reported that, relative to their premenopausal examination, those women who were perimenopausal reported 'being forgetful and having a pounding heart, hot flushes, cold sweats, constipation, joint pains and aches in the neck and/or skull'. The total number of symptoms was highest at the perimenopausal examination in those for whom longitudinal data for pre-, peri- and post-menopausal status were available.

CONSEQUENCES OF THE MENOPAUSAL TRANSITION

Cardiovascular risk factors

Very little data exist to allow an evaluation of possible changes in cardiovascular risk factors during the menopausal transition. Matthews et al (1994) reported a cohort study of 541 healthy middle-aged pre-menopausal women followed-up through the menopause. Their defini-tion of women in the perimenopause was somewhat different to that referred to in the introduction. The authors classified a woman as peri-menopausal if she reported having stopped menstruating for three months. If menses recurred she was re-classified as pre-menopausal. Thus the analysis did not specifically concentrate on a comparison of women without any change in menstrual cycle status with those who had experienced changes in flow or frequency, by self-report. Matthews et al (1994) noted no change in cardiovascular risk factors other than a small change in their levels of triglycerides for pre-menopausal women who became perimenopausal according to their definition, though they did note a marked increase in symptom reporting. Other longitudinal studies have amply confirmed adverse changes in cardiovascular risk factors when post-menopausal women are compared with their pre-menopausal counterparts, or in longitudinal studies when post-menopausal levels are compared with those prior to the final menstrual period (Jensen et al, 1990).

It seems likely that adverse changes in cardiovascular risk factors may occur as a result purely of increasing age, which could of course reflect some subtle decline in oestradiol values even in those women not yet experiencing any change in their menstrual cycle. In women at markedly increased risk of cardiovascular disease, it seems appropriate to consider oestrogen supplementation very early in the menopausal transition to minimize changes in cardiovascular risk.

Changes in bone mineral density (BMD)

There are few studies of bone loss or bone turnover in perimenopausal women. However, Gambacciani et al (1994) and Nilas and Christiansen (1989) reported radial bone loss in oligomenorrhoeic pre-menopausal women associated with an increase in FSH and bone turnover and a parallel decrease in oestradiol levels in the former but not the latter study. Slemenda et al (1987) also reported radial bone loss in late peri and post-menopausal women but not in early perimenopausal women. Mean serum oestrogen and osteocalcin concentrations predicted rates of bone loss in these women. Recent, and as yet unpublished, data from the Melbourne Mid-Life Project have shown a decrease in BMD with age in the group of perimenopausal women who also had increased levels of bone turnover markers. Again it is recommended that women at markedly increased risk of osteoporotic fracture should be considered for active intervention early in the meno-pausal transition.

CONCLUSIONS

The menopausal transition is characterized by hormonal changes associated with a period of rapid decline in ovarian follicle numbers. Marked hormonal fluctuations are observable in individual subjects and there is a substantial increase in FSH levels as menstrual irregularity occurs. Levels of oestradiol and immunoreactive inhibin in the follicular phase of the cycle change relatively little until late in the menopausal transition. The rising FSH levels presumably reflect some decline in overall oestradiol and/or inhibin and this in turn may give rise to subtle changes in lipids and BMD which are more dramatic once the final menstrual period occurs.

Characterization of an individual woman as being in the menopausal transition depends on the taking of an appropriate history, as hormonal markers are misleading and unreliable (Burger, 1994). The menopausal transition is a time when medical practitioners should be ready to provide hormonal supplementation to alleviate symptoms and to minimize adverse changes in risk factors for cardiovascular disease and osteoporosis.

SUMMARY

The menopausal transition is that period beginning with the first indications of the approach of menopause and ending with the final menses. Its morphological basis is a rapidly declining number of primordial follicles within the ovary; a decline which appears to result from an increased rate of follicular atresia. The most characteristic hormonal change in the menopausal transition is a progressive, though often fluctuating, rise in the level of serum FSH. Oestradiol and inhibin levels fluctuate markedly when observed in individual subjects but remain relatively preserved during the follicular phase of the cycle, until late in the menopausal transition. The frequency of anovulatory cycles increases as the final menstrual period approaches. The rate of symptom reporting varies among different populations of women, with maximum symptom frequency being seen during the menopausal transition. There are some indications that cardiovascular and osteoporosis risk factors may change adversely during the menopausal transition and medical practitioners should be ready to offer hormonal supplementation to women at increased risk of cardiovascular disease and osteoporotic fracture.

REFERENCES

Ahmed Ebbiary NA, Lenton EA & Cooke ID (1994) Hypothalamic-pituitary ageing: progressive increase in FSH and LH concentrations throughout the reproductive life in regularly menstruating women. *Clinical Endocrinology* **41:** 199–206.
Burger HG (1992) Inhibin. *Reproductive Medicine Review* **1:** 1–20.
Burger HG (1993) Clinical Review—Clinical utility of inhibin measurements. *Journal of Clinical Endocrinology and Metabolism* **76:** 1391–1396.
Burger HG (1994) Diagnostic role of follicle-stimulating hormone (FSH) measurements during the

menopausal transition—an analysis of FSH, oestradiol and inhibin. *European Journal of Endocrinology* **130:** 38–42.

Burger HG, Dudley EC, Hopper JL et al (1995) The endocrinology of the menopausal transition: a cross-sectional study of a population-based sample. *Journal of Clinical Endocrinology and Metabolism* **80:** 3537–3545.

Dennerstein L, Smith AM, Morse C et al (1993) Menopausal symptoms in Australian women. *Medical Journal of Australia* **259:** 232–236.

Doring GK (1969) The incidence of anovular cycles in women: *Journal of Reproduction and Fertility* **6:** 77–81.

Faddy MJ & Gosden RG (1995) A mathematical model of follicle dynamics in the human ovary. *Human Reproduction* **10:** 770–775.

Gambacciani M, Spinetti A, Taponeco F et al (1994) Bone loss in perimenopausal women: a longitudinal study. *Maturitas* **18:** 191–197.

Groome NP, Illingworth PJ, O'Brien M et al (1994) Detection of dimeric inhibin throughout the human menstrual cycle by two-site enzyme immunoassay. *Clinical Endocrinology* **40:** 717–723.

Hee J, MacNaughton J, Bangah M & Burger HG (1993) Perimenopausal patterns of gonadotrophins, immunoreactive inhibin, oestradiol and progesterone. *Maturitas* **18:** 9–20.

Hunter M, Battersby R & Whitehead M (1986) Relationships between psychological symptoms, somatic complaints and menopausal status. Maturitas **8:** 217–228.

Illingworth PJ, Reddi K, Smith KB & Baird DT (1991) The source of inhibin secretion during the human menstrual cycle. *Journal of Clinical Endocrinology and Metabolism* **73:** 667–673.

Jensen J, Nilas L & Christiansen C (1990) Influence of menopause on serum lipids and lipoproteins. *Maturitas* **12:** 321–331.

Lee SJ, Lenton EA, Sexon L & Cooke ID (1988) The effect of age on the cyclical patterns of plasma LH, FSH, oestradiol and progesterone in women with regular menstrual cycles. *Human Reproduction* **3:** 851–855.

McKinlay SM, Brambilla DJ & Posner JG (1992) The normal menopause transition. *Maturitas* **14:** 102–115.

McLachlan RI, Robertson DM, Healy DL, et al (1987) Circulating immunocreactive inhibin levels during the normal menstrual cycle. *Journal of Clinical Endocrinology and Metabolism* **65:** 954–961.

MacNaughton J, Bangah M, McCloud P et al (1992) Age related changes in follicle stimulating hormone, luteinizing hormone, oestradiol and immunoreactive inhibin in women of reproductive age. *Clinical Endocrinology* **36:** 339–345.

Matthews KA, Wing RR, Kuller LH et al (1994) Influence of the perimenopause on cardiovascular risk factors and symptoms of middle-aged healthy women. *Archives of Internal Medicine* **154:** 2349–2355.

Metcalf MG, Donald RA & Livesey JH (1981) Pituitary-ovarian function in normal women during the menopause transition. *Clinical Endocrinology* **14:** 245–255.

Nilas L & Christiansen C (1989) The pathophysiology of peri- and postmenopausal bone loss. *British Journal of Obstetrics and Gynaecology* **96:** 580–587.

Rannevik G, Jeppsson S, Johnell O et al (1995) A longitudinal study of the perimenopausal transition: altered profiles of steroid and pituitary hormones, SHBG and bone mineral density. *Maturitas* **21:** 103–113.

Richardson SJ, Senikas V & Nelson JF (1987) Follicular depletion during the menopausal transition: Evidence for accelerated loss and ultimate exhaustion. *Journal of Clinical Endocrinology and Metabolism* **65:** 1231–1237.

Sherman BM & Korenman SG (1975) Hormonal characteristics of the human menstrual cycle throughout reproductive life. *Journal of Clinical Investigation* **55:** 699–706.

Sherman BM, Wallace RB & Treloar AE (1979) The menopausal transition: Endocrinological and epidemiological considerations. *Journal of Biosocial Science* **6 (supplement):** 19–35.

Slemenda C, Hui SL, Longcope C & Johnston CC (1987) Sex steroids and bone mass. A study of changes about the time of menopause. *Journal of Clinical Investigation* **80:** 1261–1269.

2

Premature ovarian failure

DAVID H. BARLOW

This volume on 'key issues in the menopause' considers many aspects of the menopause and its management. These are issues relevant to all women since ovarian failure eventually affects all of them. This chapter is concerned with ovarian failure occurring prematurely and its consequences. When ovarian failure is premature it raises concerns similar to those considered in the other chapters, but also others relating to the prematurity of the ovarian failure. The key issues may be divided into those relating to the origin of the failure, its progress and the management of the premature oestrogen deficiency. Each of these will be considered.

LITERATURE SEARCH

The principal literature reviewed in this chapter was obtained by electronic search using Silverplatter Medline for the period 1966–1995 inclusive. The search terms were:

1. explode 'MENOPAUSE, PREMATURE'/ALL SUBHEADINGS.
2. explode 'OVARIAN FAILURE, PREMATURE'/ALL SUBHEADINGS.
3. 'MENOPAUSE' NEAR 'PREMATURE'.
4. 'OVARIAN' NEAR 'FAILURE'.
5. 'OVARY' NEAR 'FAILURE'.

DEFINING A PREMATURE MENOPAUSE

The physiological menopause is approximately 50 years of age. Generally, the menopause has been regarded as premature when it occurs before 40 years of age but it has been argued that the disadvantages of having a physiological menopause, say under 45 years of age, are such that ovarian failure should be regarded as at sufficient risk to warrant active intervention similar to that considered for those having an early menopause.

Baillière's Clinical Obstetrics and Gynaecology—
Vol. 10, No. 3, September 1996
ISBN 0–7020–2177–6
0950–3552/96/030361 + 24 $12.00/00

OVARIAN FUNCTION IN PREMATURE OVARIAN FAILURE

The clinical presentation of impaired ovarian follicular function in the presence of high gonadotropins indicates that the woman is failing to produce a normal ovarian follicular response to the gonadotropin stimulus. The endocrine basis for this change involves not only the adequacy of ovarian oestrogen output but in addition ovarian peptide output as described by Henry Burger in his chapter on the perimenopausal transition (page 352). The finding of high gonadotropin levels does not reveal whether the problem is depletion of follicles or a resistance of follicles to stimulation. This latter category is a pathophysiologically different state since the ovaries are not lacking in follicles but the follicles fail to function. Although the two states can be differentiated by ovarian histology, there has been a trend away from performing invasive ovarian biopsy simply to discover if follicles are present; we do not currently have different treatment options depending on whether premature ovarian failure (POF) is due to the resistant ovary syndrome or to a true premature menopause.

Henry Burger has described the endocrinology of perimenopausal ovarian failure (page 351). It is, however, worthwhile considering what information is available on POF.

Cameron et al (1988) reported on what may be an early stage in this failure. They studied 10 women with infertility, regular menses, and elevated follicle stimulating hormone (FSH) concentrations. The elevated FSH was not associated with significant changes in oestradiol or progesterone, but an increase in luteinizing hormone (LH) concentrations was found on some days. Plasma inhibin concentrations were normal. Subsequent assessment revealed persistently elevated FSH concentrations in 63% of the women. They considered these women to have occult ovarian failure, a condition of compensated granulosa cell function and a possible early stage of POF. Ahmed Ebbiary et al (1994) studied a similar group. They reported significantly slower follicular growth, smaller follicle diameter and lower luteal phase salivary progesterone. In both studies the prevalence of autoimmune antibodies was significantly higher in the elevated FSH groups.

Once ovarian failure is apparently established there is still a possibility that activity may occur sporadically. Rebar et al (1982) studied 26 women, under 35 years of age, with presumptive POF based on an FSH level >40 mlU/ml in karyotypically normal women with irregular menses or amenorrhoea. Nine of 18 patients had hormonal evidence of functioning ovarian follicles, and four of nine women had viable oocytes on biopsy. Evidence of ovulation was noted in five patients, and spontaneous pregnancy occurred in one. Similarly, Nelson et al (1994) studied 65 women with POF of whom nearly 50% demonstrated ovarian follicular activity, however only 16% achieved an ovulatory serum progesterone. Biopsy revealed luteinized Graafian follicles in all cases, accounting for at least 60% of the antral structures present.

The transient nature of 'ovarian failure' was emphasized by O'Herlihy et al (1980) who studied the progress of 67 women, aged under 35 years, with oligomenorrhoea or secondary amenorrhoea in whom serum FSH values were greater than 20 U/l. Twenty-four patients remained amenorrhoeic, but 17 ovulated and six conceived. The degree of increase in FSH did not correlate well with later ovarian function.

Histological studies of ovaries in POF have attempted a morphological description of the processes. Russell et al (1982) reported histology in 19 cases. In 74% the ovaries showed an absence of primordial follicles and 16% showed primordial follicles but there was little or no follicular development; this could be classed as 'resistant ovary syndrome'. Eleven per cent showed florid chronic perifollicular inflammatory reactions in the presence of both primordial and developing follicles. In a review of 10 cases by Haidar et al (1994), 80% had no follicles but in 20% follicles were present.

Mehta et al (1992) showed that vaginal ultrasound can be employed to identify a subgroup of the POF population in whom ovarian activity is continuing to some extent; 46% of POF patients had identifiable follicles. They argue that this subgroup represents those with some potential for fertility and that they may represent resistant ovary syndrome.

CAUSES OF POF

Whilst not common, POF is by no means rare in specialist practice. A survey of American women reported an age-specific incidence of 0.1% by 30 years of age and 1% by 40 years of age (Coulam et al, 1986).

Why might a woman have POF? For many we fail to identify a cause but there is a growing literature concerned with the causes.

Chromosomal anomalies

There have been a number of cytogenetic surveys of women with POF seeking detectable abnormalities. McDonough et al (1977) studied 82 women with POF and reported sex chromosome anomalies in 52 (63%). They noted that some oestrogen production was more likely to be detected if the chromosomes were normal (40%) than if there was a chromosomal anomaly (12%). In those with a genetic basis for POF, it will often result from a new mutation in that individual but there are examples of familial premature failure. Mattison et al (1984) studied five families in which a genetic association for POF was strongly suggested. Transmission was either autosomal or (less likely) X-linked dominant.

We still have only a rudimentary understanding of the chromosomal mechanisms involved in POF. In mice, Pellas et al (1991) developed an insertional transgenic mutant with abnormal germ cell development. The mouse has a recessive mutation in which both sexes have infertility and appears to affect only the reproductive organs. There is germ cell depletion from early in embryonic development without an apparent effect on somatic cells. These authors suggest that the mutated locus must play an important role in the migration or proliferation of primordial germ cells to the embryonic genital ridges.

Fragile X syndromes

Conway et al (1995) have observed a variety of fragile X permutations in familial POF. Cronister et al (1991) reported 105 heterozygous fragile X females and 90 controls. Heterozygotes and controls were divided into those with cognitive impairment (IQ less than 85) and normal IQ (IQ greater than or equal to 85). Premature menopause was present in eight of 61 normal IQ heterozygotes and in none of the impaired heterozygotes.

X-chromosome anomalies

Studies of women with POF have shown that a minority have X-chromosome anomalies, often mosaicism. Wu et al (1993) studied 61 women with POF; X-chromosome mosaicism was found in five individuals (8.2%). Other patterns seen were a complex X-chromosome mosaicism (45,X/46,XX/47,XXX), mosaic Turner's syndrome (45,X/46,XX), and mosaic triple-X syndrome (46,XX/47,XXX). They observed that the ratio of mosaic cell lines did not correlate closely with the phenotypic manifestations. Using a similar approach, Castillo et al (1992) studied 47 women with POF by cytogenetic analysis, of whom 68% had a normal karyotype. Although catalogued as normal, 11% had a 45,X cell on the karyotype. Mosiacism was identified in 15% of the women in which one cell line was normal but the other cell line involved abnormal X-chromosome patterns such as 45,X, 47,XXXX or 48,XXXX. Two cases had an abnormal chromosomal constitution 47,XXX. One young woman was found to have a reciprocal balanced translocation 46,X t(X; 18) (q21.2; q22).

Although it is possible that these translocations may lead to ovarian dysfunction by disrupting normal meiosis, the authors reinforced the concept that the study of balanced X-autosome translocation with DNA techniques could lead to identification of the gene involved in the ovarian failure by the detection of the site of disruption. This approach has been used by Powell et al (1994) who identified a patient with POF and a balanced X-autosome translocation. They used high-resolution cytogenetic analysis and flourscence in situ hybridization (FISH) to identify the translocation as 46,X,t(X;6)(q13.3 or q21;p12). They showed that her normal X was late-replicating and her translocated X earlier-replicating which is typical of balanced X-autosome rearrangements. The breakpoint was on Xq. Using a range of probes they studied DNA from the patient, her chromosomally normal parents and brother, and somatic cell hybrids containing each translocation chromosome. The translocation was found to be of paternal origin and was localized to Xq13.3-proximal Xq21.1, between PGK1 and DXS447 loci. It appears that the Xq13–q26 region is important for the achievement of normal ovarian function.

In addition, there are a number of case reports linking X-chromosome anomalies with POF. Garcia et al (1977) reported a 5/X translocation in a case of POF. Other examples of a correlation of POF with X-chromosome anomalies come from Bates and Howard (1990) who reported distal long arm deletions of the X-chromosome in POF, and Krauss et al (1987) who reported a partial deletion of the long arm of the X-chromosome (Xq) in four women of a family in which three experienced POF between the ages of 24 and 37 years. Kleczkowska et al (1993) reported a 24-year-old mentally normal female with spastic paraparesis and premature menopause showing a duplication of Xq22.3–>q27.3. Veneman et al (1991) described a family in which both the mother and her infertile daughter had premature menopause at the ages of 31 and 28 years, respectively. Initially, an extensive investigation revealed no apparent cause for their conditions. However, when cytogenetic analysis was performed in the daughter, a terminal deletion in the long arm of one of the X-chromosomes was found. The karyotype was: 46,Xdel(X),(q25-qter). Chromosomal investigation of the mother showed an identical deletion. The karyotype of the patient's 35-year-old sister is normal. She has a normal menstrual cycle and two normal children. The presence of such familial cases suggests that chromosomal investigation should be considered in young women with oligomenorrhoea, especially in those whose mothers have experienced a premature menopause.

Our understanding of the mechanisms whereby an X-chromosomal anomaly may affect the risk of POF remains vague. Fitzgerald et al (1984) hypothesized that germ cell attrition in the human female is influenced by genes of multiple effect which are carried on the X-chromosome. The more of these genes which are intact the slower the rate of germ cell attrition. More specifically, Fryns et al (1983), following the study of a 30-year-old female with symptoms of premature menopause, suggested that one mechanism was asymmetrical replication of a region on the X-chromosome with an inactive centromere, with the region of the inactive centromere replicating late. More recently, Therman and Susman (1990), noting that a lack of Xp, and especially Xcen-Xp11 (b region), in one X-chromosome may cause full-blown Turner's syndrome, have suggested that the b region (Xcen-p11) always stays active in a normal inactive X, but is inactivated in deleted X-chromosomes. This contrasts with the lack of any symptoms where truly inactivated regions of the X-chromosome are deleted. Full chromosome pairing seems to be a prerequisite for the viability of oocytes and thus for gonadal development. Deleted X-chromosomes necessarily leave a portion of the normal X unpaired and isodicentrics probably interfere with pairing, resulting in atresia of oocytes.

Other inherited conditions

Chondrodystrophy

Chondrodystrophies are a collection of inherited skeletal disorders giving short stature. Women with these conditions frequently have gynaecological problems. In particular, achondroplasia is associated with an increased risk of leiomyomata and POF (Allanson and Hall, 1986).

Galactosaemia

Another genetic mechanism which may mediate POF is the inherited autosomal recessive condition galactosaemia (galactose-1-phosphate uridyl transferase deficiency). Women homozygous for galactosaemia are at high risk of POF at an early age, but the mechanism is not fully understood; Waggoner et al (1990) surveyed a large series of cases and confirmed this high risk. Classical galactosaemia is associated with a number of long-term complications of which the most important is poor mental development. It is possible, as suggested by animal studies (Gibson 1995), that prenatal or postnatal toxicity of galactose and its metabolites causes toxic gonadal damage so that the mechanism would be follicle depletion. The use of dietary restriction is normally inadequate to prevent POF. There is evidence that the ovarian damage in galactosaemia may involve both follicle resistance and ovarian failure with the follicle resistance preceding the failure (Fraser et al, 1986).

Autoimmune abnormality

Autoimmune mechanisms are recognized as being responsible for failure in several endocrine glands including the thyroid, the adrenal and the ovary. The subject of polyendocrine autoimmunity has recently been reviewed by Weetman (1995). Reviews of women with chromosomally competent POF shows that autoimmunity can be demonstrated in approximately 40% (Alper and Garner, 1985; Belvisi et al, 1993) whereas autoantibodies are much less common in women with normal reproductive function, for example 3.6% (Belvisi et al, 1993). In a study which included chromosomally abnormal cases, Muechler et al (1991) found autoantibodies in the serum of six of 17 patients. The targets for immune reactivity included vessel walls, ovarian stromal components, follicular epithelium and antinuclear antibodies.

Our understanding of the mechanisms involved in autoimmune damage responsible for POF is improving. Dysregulation of T-lymphocyte activity appears to be involved, but the results are not consistent with those of Mignot et al (1989) who reported an increase in T-cells and especially T-helper cells in the serum of women with POF. However, Giglio et al (1994) have more recently shown that women with POF have a lower percentage of helper $CD4^+$ T-lymphocytes, higher percentages of cytotoxic $CD8^+$ T-lymphocytes and NK cells than fertile women of the same age. A reduced CD4:CD8 ratio in POF has also been reported by Ho et al (1988). In another study, Rabinowe et al (1989) did not find an increase in the CD4:CD8 ratio but they did identify some women who had elevated percentages of the specific T-lymphocyte subset characterized as 3G5+, and 35% had Ia+ (Dr activation). A potential difficulty in the interpretation of such data is the possibility that the oestrogen deficiency itself influences the balance of immune cell types (Ho et al, 1993). In functional studies, Hoek et al (1993) demonstrated dysfunction of monocytes and dendritic cells in women with POF.

Rabinowe et al (1989) also observed anti-ovarian steroid cell antibodies and anti-adrenal cortical antibodies in approximately 9% of cases. Ahonen et al (1987) showed that in women with autoimmune polyglandular disease type I, steroid cell antibodies preceded ovarian failure in all cases who subsequently developed ovarian failure but steroid cell antibodies were also found in many who did not. The sensitivity and specificity of steroid cell antibodies in predicting ovarian failure were 1.0 and 0.5, respectively. The potential use of steroid cell antibodies as a marker for potential ovarian failure has also been reported by Betterle et al (1993).

It is possible that interferon gamma, produced by activated T-lymphocytes, may play a role in autoimmunity by inducing the expression of class II major histocompatibility complex (MHC) molecules on granulosa cells thus causing the presentation of granulosa cell antigens to helper T-lymphocytes. Hill et al (1990) investigated this possibility, studying the expression of class II MHC antigens in ovaries from normal women of reproductive age and from women with autoimmune POF. Tissue from the normal women revealed minimal class II MHC expression and not on granulosa cells, whereas tissue from the autoimmune POF cases showed extensive and intense class II MHC antigen expression on granulosa cells. They also showed that, in granulosa cell cultures, class II MHC antigen expression could be induced and class I MHC antigen expression enhanced after the addition of interferon gamma.

McNatty et al (1975) showed that sera from patients with Addison's disease and ovarian dysfunction contained antibodies which reacted in vitro with human corpus luteum some of which were cytotoxic to granulosa cells in culture.

In considering the evidence on the presence of autoantibodies, it is important to emphasize that cross-reactivities frequently occur and that even where an antibody appears to be specific it is often uncertain whether the antibody has the expected action in an individual. This was emphasized by Gleicher et al (1993).

Antibodies to granulosa cell components

Winqvist et al (1995) attempted to identify the antigens on steroid-secreting cells which are associated with the immune reactivity seen in polyendocrine autoimmunity. They have recently identified the cytochrome P450 enzyme, 21-hydroxylase, and the side-chain cleavage enzyme (SCC) as the major adrenal autoantigens in Addison's disease and the autoimmune polyendocrine syndrome type I (APS-I), respectively. Since autoimmune adrenal insufficiency is associated with POF in 10 to 20% of cases, they tested sera from individuals with Addison's disease and APS-I against human granulosa cells and showed the sera to be reactive against a 51 kDa autoantigen present in granulosa cells as well as against SCC, suggesting that these may be the granulosa cell epitopes responsible for the autoimmunity.

Antibodies to zona pellucida

Smith and Hosid (1994) showed that granulosa cells may not be the only target for autoimmune reactions. They reported two cases of POF associated with antibodies directed against the zona pellucida. Whilst these studies of autoimmune reactivity by ovarian tissue are important, Wheatcroft et al (1994) suggested that some caution is needed in interpretation since they provide evidence for considerable cross-reactivity of antibodies in the sera of POF cases, having observed reactivity in 60% of sera against an ovarian biopsy and similar binding to bovine fallopian tube tissue in an enzyme-linked immunosorbent assay. It is possible that a T-cell mediated mechanism may be more important in zona pellucida immunity as a mechanism for autoimmune damage. Rhim et al (1992) demonstrated that a zona pellucida peptide from mouse ZP3 induces a CD4[+] T-cell response which mediates oophoritis.

Gonadotropin-receptor antibodies

Another potential autoimmune mechanism would be the interference of gonadotropin action by autoimmune reaction with the gonadotropin receptors. So far evidence is lacking that these autoantibodies are of significance in human POF. Tang and Farman (1983) found that gonadotropin-receptor antibodies were not more common in women with POF than in pre-menopausal and post-menopausal controls. Similarly, Anasti et al (1995) did not detect inhibitory antibodies in any of 38 POF patients. Contrary evidence is provided by van Weissenbruch et al (1991) who detected immunoglobulins that block in vitro FSH stimulated granulosa cell growth in a reasonable proportion of cases. However, considering the evidence overall, it is likely that if blocking antibodies do interfere with gonadotropin-receptor interaction as a cause of POF, it is likely they account for a small minority of cases.

Autoimmune oophoritis

The autoimmune reaction may develop to give autoimmune oophoritis as a rare cause of POF. In such patients there appears to be a marked inflammatory infiltrate and the ovary may be multicystic. In a series of 12 cases reported by Bannatyne et al (1990), eight presented as POF and four were found after gynaecological surgery. The women displayed a variety of anti-endocrine organ antibodies but most did not have anti-ovarian antibodies. There was an inflammatory infiltrate which spared primordial follicles but involved pre-ovulatory follicles and corpora lutea and there were peri-vascular and perineural inflammatory infiltrates. The inflammatory infiltrate included humoral and cellular immune elements characterized as B cells, plasma cells, T-cells and macrophages (Sedmak et al, 1987). Lonsdale et al (1991) reviewed the presence of cysts in autoimmune oophoritis, reporting them in five of 17 cases and emphasized the importance of recognizing the condition because it is associated with a high risk of Addison's disease. Biscotti et al (1989) warned that women with cystic expression of autoimmune oophoritis are at risk of unnecessary surgical intervention and losing ovarian tissue when their ovarian function is already compromised.

Cancer therapy and POF

A well recognized cause of POF is ovarian 'damage' as a result of exposure to radiotherapy or chemotherapy as treatment for malignant disease. The potential for POF will be influenced by a number of variables including reproductive status and age at treatment, the exposure to therapy, and the condition being treated which is the major determinant of the treatment modality.

Mechanisms of chemotherapeutic damage

The mechanism of the damage brought about by cancer therapy has been examined in a number of animal studies. The principle agent studied has been cyclophosphamide, an alkylating drug with the most prominent ovarian toxicity in common use. Shiromozu et al (1984) showed that destruction of primordial follicles occurs quickly, with medium sized follicles damaged after a few days exposure and large follicles after several weeks. In an in vitro rat granulosa cell system, Ramahi Ataya et al (1988) demonstrated this toxicity at concentrations as low as $10\,\mu g/ml$. Using rat oocyte in vitro fertilisation as a model for cyclophosphamide treatment, interference with the fertilising function of oocytes was shown (Ataya et al, 1988; Pydyn and Ataya, 1991). Again, in a rat granulosa cell system at concentrations lower than those used in chemotherapy, vinblastine has been shown to interfere with in vitro production of progesterone and prostaglandin E (Teaff et al, 1990). The detailed mechanisms are not yet understood, however, recently Cusido et al (1995) demonstrated that cyclophosphamide increases the frequency of synaptonemal complex and nucleolar fragmentation in proliferating rat germ cells.

Breast cancer

The management of breast cancer may involve adjuvant chemotherapy and/or long-term tamoxifen treatment. Studies by Reichman and Green (1994) recently reviewed the literature on the reproductive effects of chemotherapy for breast cancer. Cyclophosphamide is a major cause of POF which may occur. They noted that the degree of ovarian dysfunction was related to age, dose and duration of treatment.

In a study of 131 pre-menopausal women on adjuvant chemotherapy for breast cancer, Samaan et al (1978) showed that 71% became amenorrhoeic and demonstrated that the amenorrhoea was due to ovarian failure. A similar risk was reported by Hortobagyi et al (1986) with 80% of a large series of breast cancer cases given doxorubicin developing amenorrhoea.

There was a clear age effect with none of the patients under 30 years of age having menstrual abnormalities, whereas 96% of those 40 to 49 years of age developed amenorrhoea. Amenorrhoea was permanent for most women over 40 years of age, but for 50% of patients under 40, it was reversible. Bhatavdekar et al (1992) showed that the cumulative dose of breast cancer adjuvant chemotherapy was relevant to the risk of ovarian damage, with amenorrhoea occurring within two to five months in older patients; younger patients required large cumulative doses of cytotoxic drugs to exhibit ovarian dysfunction. In a randomized controlled trial comparing 12 and 36 weeks of stage II breast cancer chemotherapy (Reyno et al, 1992), the overall rate of inducing amenorrhoea in pre-menopausal women was 71% with a statistically significant difference between the short (55%) and long (83%) exposure groups. Interestingly, these authors reported that the disease recurrence rate was significantly lower in those who became amenorrhoeic than in those who did not; 38 versus 57%. The effect of induced-amenorrhoea on outcome was seen predominantly in patients under 40 years of age. This age sensitivity is further emphasized by Koyama et al (1977) who observed that the average total dose of cyclophosphamide associated with the induction of amenorrhoea in breast cancer cases is higher in women in their 30s (9.3 g) than in their 40s (5.2 g).

When tamoxifen is included in the chemotherapeutic regimen, the endocrinology becomes more complex but this is not necessarily to the patient's disadvantage since the additional effect relates to the partial oestrogen agonist action of tamoxifen. In an endocrine study comparing responses to adjuvant chemotherapy alone or in combination with tamoxifen, Jordan et al (1987) found that ovarian failure which occurred in a group receiving tamoxifen was not associated with the rise in gonadotropins which is expected in ovarian failure and which was observed in the other treatment group. When the tamoxifen is stopped, the gonadotropins then rise into the post-menopausal range. Thus there is a need for caution in the interpretation of gonadotropin levels in women on tamoxifen who are concerned that their chemotherapy might have damaged their ovaries and are requesting assessment.

Lymphoma

Women with lymphoma (Hodgkin's disease (HD) and non-Hodgkin's lymphoma (NHL)), may be exposed to chemotherapy or radiotherapy and may be younger on average than breast cancer patients. A particularly detailed study was reported by Chapman et al (1979) in which pre-treatment ovarian biopsies were taken to confirm ovarian normality before therapy. They assigned 41 cases after therapy to one of three categories: POF (49%), irregular ovarian activity (34%), and normal ovarian activity (17%). In 16 months, a progressive loss of ovarian function occurred that was clearly age-related but not statistically dose-related. This age effect has also been reported by Schilsky et al (1981), Whitehead et al (1983), Kreuser et al (1987) and Fisher and Cheung (1984).

Fisher and Cheung (1984) studied 51 women and found that the most favourable prognosis was associated with young age at primary treatment, especially pre-menarchal, and irradiation confined to above the pelvic brim, whereas in those women over 40 years of age who were exposed to irradiation below the pelvic brim, there was a high probability of ovarian failure. Overall, 55% of female patients under the age of 50 treated with chemotherapy alone or with radiation therapy above the pelvic brim retained normal ovarian function. Kreuser et al (1987) studied 14 women who had quadruple chemotherapy and reported permanent ovarian failure in 57%. The incidence of ovarian failure in women over 24 years of age was 86% versus 28% in those under 24 years. Whitehead et al (1983) studied 44 women who had previously received quadruple chemotherapy with long-term follow-up (median, 30 months). Regular menses continued in 39%, whereas 23% developed oligomenorrhoea and 39% amenorrhoea. Those who subsequently developed amenorrhoea were significantly older (median, 30 years) than those who maintained regular menses (median, 22 years) or developed oligomenorrhoea (median, 23 years). Schilsky et al (1981) studied 27 women given quadruple chemotherapy, some with additional extrapelvic radiotherapy, with an even longer follow-up (median, nine years) and median age of 30. Persistent amenorrhoea occurred in 46%, 89% of whom were older than 25 at the time of treatment. In contrast, 80% of patients younger than 25 at treatment continued to menstruate regularly.

Specht et al (1984) reported on a series of 16 young women restricted to combination therapy for less advanced disease. Ovarian failure occurred in 25% whereas ovarian function continued in 75%, 67% of whom achieved pregnancy. Again, those with ovarian failure tended to be older. They concluded that for women under 35 years of age, the long-term chances of preserving ovarian function after standard treatment for the early stages of HD is good. Recent studies have reported similar findings in early stage disease (Madsen et al, 1995) and with a low-dose approach in young women (Hudson et al, 1993). Another potential factor in ovarian prognosis is the type of lymphoma since the different forms may involve different patterns of therapy. Bokemeyer et al (1994) studied relapse-free survivors with high-grade NHL or with HD who were under 45 years of age. Only 10% of the NHL group but 50% of the HD group showed signs of ovarian failure. This latter group was exposed to higher cumulative doses of both procarbazine and more intense radiotherapy.

Leukaemia

The leukaemias and related blood dyscrasias are another category of malignant disease which may commonly affect women of reproductive age, and may also affect adolescents or pre-pubertal girls. Treatment generally involves chemotherapy and/or radiotherapy and bone marrow transplant. In a detailed study, Sanders et al (1988) studied 187 women between 13 and 49 years of age from one to 15 years (median, four years) after marrow transplant for aplastic anaemia or leukaemia. Among 43 women transplanted for aplastic anaemia, ovarian failure occurred in 69% of those over

26 years of age but in none below that age. Of 144 women transplanted for leukaemia, only 6% recovered ovarian function. Both total body irradiation (TBI) and greater patient age were significantly associated with a decreased probability of recovering normal ovarian function. By seven years after transplant, the probabilities of having normal ovarian function were 0.92 after cyclophosphamide chemotherapy alone and 0.24 after cyclophosphamide plus TBI. This poor prognosis for ovarian function after TBI used in adults is emphasized in another large follow-up study by Spinelli et al (1994) who reported most of 79 women receiving TBI as having a premature menopause with 94% of sexually active women reporting sexual difficulties following treatment. In smaller studies, Benker et al (1989) and Keilholz et al (1989) reported ovarian failure in all women treated. Where the treatment of leukaemia occurs in childhood there is a risk of hypothalamic–pituitary damage with effects on the dependent endocrine axes. However, there is also a risk of pre-pubertal ovarian damage leading to ovarian failure as reported in 12% of a series reported by Shalet et al (1977).

Other cancers

The literature on other cancers and the risk of ovarian failure is limited. A follow-up study on 22 women treated for choriocarcinoma (Choo et al, 1985) indicated that seven (39%) experienced ovarian failure, yet in all but two of the cases, who were older, the failure was transient. Raymond et al (1989) reported that radioiodine therapy for thyroid cancer may be associated with temporary ovarian failure during the first year after treatment, the risk being 27% in that study.

Lupus nephritis

Radiotherapy or chemotherapy may also be given for the management of lupus nephritis which is not responding to steroid therapy. Strober et al (1985) reported a case of ovarian failure in a woman managed with lymphoid radiotherapy and Ginzler et al (1976) demonstrated ovarian failure where cyclophosphamide was added to a drug regimen.

Childhood cancer

Children may be exposed to abdominal radiotherapy for a number of cancer indications. In a large follow-up study of 182 long-term survivors of childhood malignancy, Stillman et al (1981) found that 12% had ovarian failure. The position of the ovaries in relation to the radiotherapy field was an important factor, with ovarian failure occurring in 68% of those who had both ovaries within the abdominal radiotherapy field, in 14% of those whose ovaries were at the edge of the field, and in none of those with one or both ovaries outside the field. The odds for ovarian failure in patients with both ovaries in the field are 19.7 higher than those for other irradiated patients. Similarly, Wallace et al (1989) found that, of 53 survivors of childhood abdominal tumours, whole abdominal radiotherapy was associated with a premature menopause in 26% and some degree of pubertal failure in 71%. Where flank radiotherapy was used, only 7% had pubertal failure and none subsequently had premature menopause.

Minimizing ovarian damage

Since the ovarian consequences of cancer therapy can be so serious attention has focused on strategies which might minimize the risk of ovarian failure. On the basis that inactive follicles might be less susceptible to damage, there has been interest in temporarily inducing ovarian inactivity via gonadotropin-releasing hormone (GnRH) agonist therapy during cancer treatment. Another strategy has been the surgical transposition of the ovaries prior to radiotherapy.

In a study of GnRH agonist suppression of follicular activity in monkeys, Ataya et al (1995) found that ovarian failure due to radiation was not prevented by this strategy. They were able to examine follicle counts and reported that the GnRH agonist did not prevent the follicle depletion caused by irradiation. More promising results were obtained by Montz et al (1991), who used a rat model in which cyclophosphamide chemotherapy was given alone or opposed by a progesterone or a GnRH agonist. They found that progesterone was able to protect the gonad, maintaining fertility and fecundity rates not significantly different from those of the untreated control animals. The GnRH agonist had a similar effect on fertility, but failed to protect fecundity.

The aim of surgical transposition of the ovaries is to place them as far out of the main radiation field as is possible in women about to have radiotherapy. Van Beurden et al (1990) showed that with this approach at least one ovary can be placed outside the radiation field in 68% of cases but because of scattered radiation a substantial loss of ovarian function might still occur. In a study of ovarian transposition during surgery for stage II cervical cancer (Owens et al, 1989), none of 14 women developed ovarian failure. In a much larger study, Feeney et al (1995) reviewed 132 cases of stage I-IIA cervical cancer treated primarily with radical hysterectomy and pelvic lymphadenectomy in whom lateral ovarian transposition was performed. Twenty-eight of these women received post-operative pelvic radiotherapy; only three (2.9%) of those who did not have radiotherapy experienced menopausal symptoms, and FSH levels suggested that they did not have ovarian failure. However, ovarian failure occurred in 14 (50%) women who received post-operative pelvic radiation therapy thus the procedure did not protect all women although the proportion affected was likely to be lower than expected. Williams and Mendenhall (1992) reported a laparoscopic technique which might be used to displace the ovaries away from the pelvic nodal area in women about to have pelvic radiotherapy, without incurring delays from laparotomy when primary treatment does not require surgery.

Post-hysterectomy ovarian failure

A woman who has a hysterectomy loses the principal marker of continuing ovarian function; the menstrual period. She can only judge the onset of the menopause by the start of menopausal symptoms or by the measurement of elevated plasma FSH. Since these parameters often precede the menopause in non-hysterectomized women, they are not exact markers of the menopause but do approximate to ovarian failure. If women who have hysterectomy involving the conservation of one or both ovaries are at risk of an earlier menopause then, for the reasons stated, this may go undetected if symptoms are not prominent. Again, for these reasons, it has been difficult to determine the degree of risk of a 'premature menopause' after conservative hysterectomy, although in surveys of menopausal symptoms, hysterectomized women seem to experience more problems than non-hysterectomized ones (Sessums and Murphy, 1932; Barlow et al, 1989; Seidenschnur et al, 1989; Oldenhave et al, 1993). Using secondary measures of oestrogen production such as vaginal cytology, Bancroft-Livingstone (1954) concluded that hysterectomy did not hasten the onset of the menopause, whereas both Whitelaw (1958) and de Neef and Hollenbeck (1966) concluded from cytology that although oestrogen production continued, ovulation occurred in only about a quarter to a third of hysterectomized women.

More direct evidence was provided by the histology of retained ovaries subsequently removed at laparotomy (Grogan, 1958). Corpora lutea were found in 50% of ovaries and developing follicles in 10% giving an overall prevalence of activity of 60%. In a survey employing regular urine collection to assess the levels of oestrogen and progesterone production, Beavis et al (1969) reported ovulation in 64% of cases, anovulation in 22% and ovarian failure in 14%. After radical hysterectomy for cervical carcinoma, Parker et al (1993) reported that 20% of women developed ovarian failure. Using a symptom questionnaire, Riedel et al (1986) found typical signs of ovarian failure in 39% of 164 hysterectomized women and, in a subgroup who had undergone endocrine investigation, they found ovarian activity continuing in most cases but with impaired luteal function. In another symptom survey, Menon et al (1987) found a high prevalence of hot flushes in 60 post-hysterectomy cases with endocrine investigation revealing that only 8% had ovarian failure. They did note that those who complained of hot flushes but did not have ovarian failure did have a lower mean bone mineral density (BMD) than those who did not flush, implying some degree of impaired oestrogen production short of ovarian failure.

A lower BMD in hysterectomized women was also reported by Hreshchyshyn et al (1988) and Centerwall (1981) indicated that women having pre-menopausal hysterectomy have an increased risk of cardio-vascular disease.

One difficulty in assessing the potential for subsequent problems in a hysterectomy population, is the uncertainty of problems occurring if surgery is not performed. No study has solved this dilemma, but the best one so far is that by Siddle et al (1987) who examined 90 women who had undergone abdominal hysterectomy with bilateral ovarian conservation, and 226 women who had undergone a spontaneous menopause. The mean age of ovarian failure in the hysterectomized group was significantly lower at 45.4 years compared to 49.5 years; the mean age in the control group. They found that the indication for hysterectomy did not influence the time of ovarian failure, but that there was a significant correlation between the age at hysterectomy and the age of ovarian failure in those women of 44 years of age or less at the time of ovarian failure, implying a causal relationship. This literature, despite its shortcomings, presents a picture of an above average degree of distress from problems, ovarian failure in a small proportion of cases with retained ovaries, and the possibility of premature menopause. However, we await a definitive study. Clearly, any hysterectomized woman reporting symptoms should be assessed for FSH levels regardless of how young she is.

CONSEQUENCES OF PREMATURE MENOPAUSE

Oestrogen deficiency symptoms

Cust et al (1989) reported on oestrogen deficiency symptoms in 36 women who had ovarian failure after TBI and bone marrow transplant for leukaemia. Thirty-three reported symptoms including vaginal dryness which affected sexual function, 16 a decrease in libido and 18 difficulties with sexual intercourse. Treatment seemed effective in abolishing symptoms in 24 of the women, but vaginal dryness remained a problem in three. Two women failed to respond and intercourse remained impossible. Many reported reduced self-confidence. These forms of distress were also reported in a survey of post-chemotherapy patients by Chapman et al (1979) and in post-irradiation patients by Spinelli et al (1994).

Bone loss in POF

John Kanis has described the factors controlling bone mass and the impact of oestrogen deficiency on the skeleton (page 473). Women who experience POF are therefore theoretically at increased risk of osteoporosis. Caplan et al (1994) studied 214 women with vertebral crush fractures and found that 26% had undergone a natural menopause before 45 years of age; this was more than twice as many women as had lost ovarian function early because of surgery.

Risk of low BMD

What is the risk of significant bone loss in groups of women with POF? Both Cann et al (1984) and Jones et al (1985) reported on the risk of osteoporosis in pre-menopausal amenorrhoea. Both studies showed that POF with different forms of amenorrhoea was associated with the most marked reductions in BMD compared to controls, particularly at the spine, whereas Cann et al (1984) observed a decrease in BMD of 20 to 30%. Kurabayashi et al (1993) observed that untreated POF and women with Turner's syndrome had similar low BMD levels compared to controls.

Examining only women with untreated POF and controls, Bagur and Mautalen (1992) reported obesity, which can be associated with higher circulating oestrogen levels, as a relevant factor, with four obese POF cases showing no significant loss of BMD at the spine and proximal femur compared to controls. In contrast, non-obese POF cases had significantly lower BMD compared with healthy young women, age-matched and menopause-matched controls, particularly at the lumbar spine than the proximal femur. This spinal BMD deficit correlated with the time elapsed since the start of the premature menopause. Nearly half of non-obese patients had a vertebral BMD below the fracture threshold and a quarter were below the fracture threshold for hip BMD.

Some studies have reported on bone loss in specific subgroups of POF cases; several have looked at women who received cancer therapy and one reported on POF due to galactosaemia. All suggested a reduced BMD in women with POF. Ratcliffe et al (1992) showed reduced BMD in chemotherapy-treated lymphoma survivors who had become post-menopausal, particularly with longer durations of amenorrhoea, but no reduction in those whose ovarian function had continued. Similar findings were reported for a HD cohort (Kreuser et al, 1992) and for a cohort having received adjuvant chemotherapy for pre-menopausal breast cancer (Bruning et al, 1990). A well controlled study was carried out on HD survivors all of whom had been treated at least five years earlier (Redman et al, 1988). The study included pre-menopausal and post-menopausal control groups and HD cases with and without POF. The cases with POF were subdivided into those who did, or did not, receive hormone replacement therapy (HRT). They showed that the non-HRT POF group had reduced BMD at multiple sites compared to the pre-menopausal controls, and had a similar BMD to the post-menopausal controls. The HD group without POF and the HRT POF group had BMD values generally similar to the pre-menopausal controls.

Kaufman et al (1993) studied a group of women with POF due to galactosaemia. Compared with age- and sex-matched controls, patients with galactosaemia had diminished BMD. They indicated that oestrogen deficiency is not the only factor in reduced bone mass because even pre-pubertal galactosaemic females had reduced BMD relative to controls. The use of HRT did not return BMD to normal levels but those not given HRT had even lower BMD.

HRT for prevention of bone loss

The influence of HRT on BMD in POF has been reported by several authors. In these studies, women with POF had lower BMD than controls without POF. Louis et al (1989) and Metka et al (1992) both reported that HRT produced a rise in BMD. This rise reflects the fall in bone turnover induced by the HRT and cannot be assumed to indicate that the rise would continue long-term, as discussed by John Kanis (page 472), but it does indicate the positive effect of HRT in this patient group. In studies by Soong et al (1989), Emans et al (1990) and Kurabayashi et al (1993), HRT was able to decrease the severity of bone loss, but did not increase BMD.

Oral contraceptives for prevention of bone loss

Many women with POF are at an age where their contemporaries are more likely to be familiar with oral contraceptives than with HRT. Gambacciani et al (1994) studied bone responses in 16 women entering perimenopausal ovarian failure given a low-dose oral contraceptive and demonstrated preservation of bone mass.

FERTILITY AFTER POF

Temporary ovarian failure

Generally, ovarian failure is an irreversible state but there are examples of spontaneous recovery and fertility in such cases. After autoimmune ovarian failure there are examples of spontaneous recovery even after 12 years (Taylor et al, 1989) or after the treatment of coexisting thyroid and adrenal autoimmune disease (Finer et al, 1985). Spontaneous recovery after POF induced by cancer therapy was reported by Raymond et al (1989) after radioiodine therapy for thyroid cancer and Shalev et al (1987) after busulfan-induced POF in a leukaemia patient. In an assessment of women with POF seeking oocyte donation as a means to achieve pregnancy, Kreiner et al (1988) observed ovulation in seven of 63 (11.1%) with POF; three of 63 (4.8%) conceived and delivered normal, healthy infants. They argue that women in this situation should be given a trial on oestrogen replacement with close monitoring of ovulation before oocyte donation.

Fertility therapy in POF

Although spontaneous ovarian activity may occur in women with POF, clinicians have little ability to manipulate the potential for ovarian activity and fertility. Anasti et al (1994) explored the possibility that the immunomodulatory action of danazol might be of value in managing infertility in POF but found it of no value.

The use of ovulation induction therapy in women who already show high gonadotropin levels is generally unsuccessful but there is some evidence that a minority of cases can respond. Using gonadotropin therapy in 15 women with autoimmune POF, Blumenfeld et al (1993) showed a conception rate of approximately 40% after three cycles of treatment (14 pregnancies in eight women, two of which were spontaneous). The authors emphasized that the autoimmune group appeared particularly responsive to therapy. More generally the results of ovulation induction in POF have been poor.

There has been interest in inducing gonadotropin suppression to see if this might render follicles more responsive to subsequent gonadotropin stimulation. The commonest method used has been oestrogen therapy, which can occasionally achieve the desired effect (Check et al, 1988) but is generally disappointing. Buckler et al (1993) reported that this approach did not result in normal follicular activity in eight women after release from gonadotropin suppression due to a combined oral contraceptive. In an early report by Fleming et al (1984), a pregnancy was achieved in the first cycle of gonadotropin therapy given after achieving pituitary down-regulation using a GnRH agonist in a woman with POF due to chemotherapy for HD; however, subsequent experience with this approach has been disappointing. Nelson et al (1992) in a controlled trial of 26 women and Ledger et al (1989) in a trial of 12 women reported that GnRH agonist suppression of gonadotropins did not prove effective.

Ovum donation

The slim chances that ovarian function might spontaneously return or that ovulation induction therapy might actually work, is of little help to the many women with POF who wish pregnancy. In recent years these women have, for the first time, an effective treatment option in the form of egg donation, if this is acceptable to them. Pados et al (1992) reported on a series of 336 oocyte replacement cycles in 199 patients. A clinical pregnancy rate of 34.7% per patient was achieved. The highest pregnancy rate among patients with ovarian failure was observed in those with POF (26.4%; 14/53), while the lowest was among women who had received chemotherapy and/or radiotherapy (9%; 1/11). Similar results were reported by Sauer et al (1994) in a series of 300 cycles, again reporting that those with premature menopause due to chemotherapy had a poorer performance than the other groups requiring oocyte donation. Hens et al (1989) showed that women with POF due to X-chromosomal anomalies can have the same effectiveness with oocyte donation as those with a normal 46, XX karyotype. There is little doubt that ovum donation is the effective option for women with POF who desire pregnancy and who can accept the idea of donated gametes; unfortunately the limited supply of donates oocytes remains a major problem, so that clinics offering that option have long waiting lists.

Conclusion

Women who experience a premature menopause, for whatever reason, are at risk of symptoms and long-term effects which are largely preventable by the appropriate use of HRT. They differ from older women expecting the menopause in that they are often having to face an unexpected loss of fertility in addition, and may be having to cope with concerns about cancer. It is important that the particular needs of such women are understood and met.

REFERENCES

Ahmed Ebbiary NA, Lenton EA, Salt C et al (1994) The significance of elevated basal follicle stimulating hormone in regularly menstruating infertile women. *Human Reproduction* **9:** 245–252.

Ahonen P, Miettinen A & Perheentupa J (1987) Adrenal and steroidal cell antibodies in patients with autoimmune polyglandular disease type I and risk of adrenocortical and ovarian failure. *Journal of Clinical Endocrinology and Metabolism* **64:** 494–500.

Allanson JE & Hall JG (1986) Obstetric and gynecologic problems in women with chondrodystrophies. *Obstetrics and Gynecology* **67:** 74–78.

Alper MM & Garner PR (1985) Premature ovarian failure: its relationship to autoimmune disease. *Obstetrics and Gynecology* **66:** 27–30.

Anasti JN, Flack MR, Froehlich J & Nelson LM (1995) The use of human recombinant gonadotropin receptors to search for immunoglobulin G-mediated premature ovarian failure. *Journal of Clinical Endocrinology and Metabolism* **80:** 824–828.

Anasti JN, Kimzey LM, Defensor RA et al (1994) A controlled study of danazol for the treatment of karyotypically normal spontaneous premature ovarian failure. *Fertility and Sterility* **62:** 726–730.

Ataya KM, Pydyn EF & Sacco AG (1988) Effect of 'activated' cyclophosphamide on mouse oocyte in vitro fertilization and cleavage. *Reproductive Toxicology* **2:** 105–109.

Ataya K, Pydyn E, Ramahi Ataya A & Orton CG (1995) Is radiation-induced ovarian failure in rhesus monkeys preventable by luteinizing hormone-releasing hormone agonists?: Preliminary observations. *Journal of Clinical Endocrinology and Metabolism* **80:** 790–795.

Bagur AC & Mautalen CA (1992) Risk for developing osteoporosis in untreated premature menopause. *Calcified Tissue International* **51:** 4–7.

Bancroft-Livingstone G (1954) Ovarian survival following hysterectomy. *Journal of Obstetrics and Gynaecology of the British Empire* **61:** 628–638.

Bannatyne P, Russell P & Shearman RP (1990) Autoimmune oophoritis: a clinicopathologic assessment of 12 cases. *International Journal of Gynecological Pathology* **9:** 191–207.

Barlow DH, Grosset KA, Hart H & Hart DM (1989) A study of the experience of Glasgow women in the climacteric years. *British Journal of Obstetrics and Gynaecology* **96:** 1192–1197.

Bates A & Howard PJ (1990) Distal long arm deletions of the X chromosome and ovarian failure. *Journal of Medical Genetics* **27:** 722–723.

Beavis EL, Brown JB & Smith MA (1969) Ovarian function after hysterectomy with conservation of the ovaries in pre-menopausal women. *Journal of Obstetrics and Gynaecology of the British Commonwealth* **76:** 969–978.

Belvisi L, Bombelli F, Sironi L & Doldi N (1993) Organ-specific autoimmunity in patients with premature ovarian failure. *Journal of Endocrinological Investigation* **16:** 889–892.

Benker G, Schafer U, Hermanns U et al (1989) Allogenic bone marrow transplantation in adults: endocrine sequelae after 1–6 years. *Acta Endocrinologica Copenhagen* **120:** 37–42.

Betterle C, Rossi A, Dalla Pria S et al (1993) A. Premature ovarian failure: autoimmunity and natural history. *Clinical Endocrinology Oxford.* **39:** 35–43.

Bhatavdekar JM, Shah NG, Patel DD et al (1992) Endocrine function in premenopausal and postmenopausal advanced breast cancer patients treated with CMF or tamoxifen. *Neoplasma* **39:** 123–127.

Biscotti CV, Hart WR & Lucas JG (1989) Cystic ovarian enlargement resulting from autoimmune oophoritis. *Obstetrics and Gynecology* **74:** 492–495.

Blumenfeld Z, Halachmi S, Peretz BA et al (1993) Premature ovarian failure—the prognostic application of autoimmunity on conception after ovulation induction *Fertility and Sterility* **59:** 750–755.

Bokemeyer C, Schmoll HJ, van Rhee J et al (1994) Long-term gonadal toxicity after therapy for Hodgkin's and non-Hodgkin's lymphoma. *Annals of Hematology* **68:** 105–110.

Bruning PF, Pit MJ, de Jong Bakker M, et al (1990) Bone mineral density after adjuvant chemotherapy for premenopausal breast cancer. *British Journal of Cancer* **61:** 308–310.

Buckler HM, Healy DL & Burger HG (1993) Does gonadotropin suppression result in follicular development in premature ovarian failure? *Gynecology and Endocrinology* **7:** 123–128.

Byrne J, Fears TR, Gail MH et al (1992) Early menopause in long-term survivors of cancer during adolescence. *American Journal of Obstetrics and Gynecology* **166:** 788–793.

Cameron IT, O'Shea FC, Rolland JM et al (1988) Occult ovarian failure: a syndrome of infertility, regular menses, and elevated follicle-stimulating hormone concentrations. *Journal of Clinical Endocrinology and Metabolism* **67**: 1190–1194.

Cann CE, Martin MC, Genant HK & Jaffe RB (1984) Decreased spinal, mineral content in amenorrheic women. *Journal of the American Medical Association* **251**: 626–629.

Caplan GA, Scane AC & Francis RM (1994) Pathogenesis of vertebral crush fractures in women. *Journal of the Royal Society of Medicine* **87**: 200–202.

Castillo S, Lopez F, Tobella L et al (1992) The cytogenetics of premature ovarian failure. *Revista Chilena de Obstetricia y Ginecologica* **57**: 341–345.

Centerwall BS (1981) Premenopausal hysterectomy and cardiovascular disease. *American Journal of Obstetrics and Gynecology* **139**: 58–61.

Chapman RM, Sutcliffe SB & Malpas JS (1979) Cytotoxic-induced ovarian failure in women with Hodgkin's disease. I. Hormone function. *Journal of the American Medical Association* **242**: 1877–1881.

Check JH, Wu CH & Check ML (1988) The effect of leuprolide acetate in aiding induction of ovulation in hypergonadotropic hypogonadism: a case report. *Fertility and Sterility* **49**: 542–543.

Choo YC, Chan SY, Wong LC & Ma HK (1985) Ovarian dysfunction in patients with gestational trophoblastic neoplasia treated with short intensive courses of etoposide (VP-16–213). *Cancer* **55**: 2348–2352.

Conway GS, Hettiarachchi S, Murray A & Jacobs PA (1995) Fragile X premutations in familial premature ovarian failure. *Lancet* **346**: 309–310.

Coulam CB, Adamson SC & Annegers JF (1986) Incidence of premature ovarian failure. *Obstetrics and Gynecology* **67**: 604–606.

Cronister A, Schreiner R, Wittenberger M et al (1991) Heterozygous fragile X female: historical, physical, cognitive, and cytogenetic features. *American Journal of Medical Genetics* **38**: 269–274.

Cusido L, Pujol R, Egozcue J & Garcia M (1995) Cyclophosphamide-induced synaptonemal complex damage during meiotic prophase of female *Rattus norvegicus*. *Mutation Research* **329**: 131–141.

Cust MP, Whitehead MI, Powles R et al (1989) Consequences and treatment of ovarian failure after total body irradiation for leukaemia. *British Medical Journal* **299**: 1494–1497.

de Neef JC & Hollenbeck ZJ (1966) The fate of ovaries preserved at the time of hysterectomy. *American Journal of Obstetrics and Gynecology* **96**: 1088–1097.

Emans SJ, Grace E, Hoffer FA et al (1990) Estrogen deficiency in adolescents and young adults: impact on bone mineral content and effects of estrogen replacement therapy. *Obstetrics and Gynecology* **76**: 585–592.

Feeney DD, Moore DH, Look KY et al (1995) The fate of the ovaries after radical hysterectomy and ovarian transposition. *Gynecologic Oncology* **56**: 3–7.

Finer N, Fogelman I & Bottazzo G (1985) Pregnancy in a woman with premature ovarian failure. *Postgraduate Medical Journal* **61**: 1079–1080.

Fisher B & Cheung AY (1984) Delayed effect of radiation therapy with or without chemotherapy on ovarian function in women with Hodgkin's disease. *Acta Radiologica Oncologica* **23**: 43–48.

Fitzgerald PH, Donald RA & McCormick P (1984) Reduced fertility in women with X chromosome abnormality. *Clinical Genetics* **25**: 301–309.

Fleming R, Hamilton MPR, Barlow DH et al (1984) Pregnancy after ovulation induction in a patient with menopausal gonadotrophin levels after chemotherapy. *Lancet* **i**: 399.

Fraser IS, Russell P, Greco S & Robertson DM (1986) Resistant ovary syndrome and premature ovarian failure in young women with galactosaemia. *Clinics of Reproduction and Fertility* **4**: 133–138.

Fryns JP, Petit P, Kleczkowska A & van den Berghe H (1983) Replication and inactivation of an isodicentric X: presence of an inactive centromere influences the replication patterns. *Clinical Genetics* **24**: 180–183.

Gambacciani M, Spinetti A, Cappagli B et al (1994) Hormone replacement therapy in perimenopausal women with a low dose oral contraceptive preparation: effects on bone mineral density and metabolism. *Maturitas* **19**: 125–131.

Garcia JE, Cummings DK, Wentz AC et al (1977) A 5/X chromosomal translocation in a patient with premature menopause. *Journal of Hereditary* **68**: 75–80.

Gibson JB (1995) Gonadal function in galactosemics and in galactose-intoxicated animals. *European Journal of Pediatrics* **154**: S14–S20.

Giglio T, Imro MA, Filaci G et al (1994) Immune cell circulating subsets are affected by gonadal function. *Life Science* **54**: 1305–1312.

Ginzler E, Diamond H, Guttadauria M & Kaplan D (1976) Prednisone and azathioprine compared to prednisone plus low-dose azathioprine and cyclophosphamide in the treatment of diffuse lupus nephritis. *Arthritis and Rheumatism* **19:** 693–699.

Gleicher N, Pratt D & Dudkiewicz A (1993) What do we really know about autoantibody abnormalities and reproductive failure?: a critical review. *Autoimmunity* **16:** 115–140.

Grogan RH (1958) Residual ovaries. *Obstetrics and Gynecology* **12:** 329–332.

Haidar MA, Baracat EC, Simoes MJ et al (1994) Premature ovarian failure: morphological and ultrastructural aspects. *Revista Paulista de Medicina* **112:** 534–538.

Hens L, Devroey P, Van Waesberghe L et al (1989) Chromosome studies and fertility treatment in women with ovarian failure. *Clinical Genetics* **36:** 81–91.

Hill JA, Welch WR, Faris HM & Anderson DJ (1990) Induction of class II major histocompatibility complex antigen expression in human granulosa cells by interferon gamma: a potential mechanism contributing to autoimmune ovarian failure. *American Journal of Obstetrics and Gynecology* **162:** 534–540.

Ho PC, Tang GW, Fu KH et al (1988) Immunologic studies in patients with premature ovarian failure. *Obstetrics and Gynecology* **71:** 622–626.

Ho PC, Tang GW & Lawton JW (1993) Lymphocyte subsets and serum immunoglobulins in patients with premature ovarian failure before and after oestrogen replacement. *Human Reproduction* **8:** 714–716.

Hoek A, van Kasteren Y, de Haan Meulman M et al (1993) Dysfunction of monocytes and dendritic cells in patients with premature ovarian failure. *American Journal of Reproductive Immunology* **30:** 207–217.

Hortobagyi GN, Buzdar AU, Marcus CE & Smith TL (1986) Immediate and long-term toxicity of adjuvant chemotherapy regimens containing doxorubicin in trials at M.D. Anderson Hospital and Tumor Institute. *NCI Monographs:* 105–109.

Hreshchyshyn MM, Hopkins A, Zylstra S & Anbar M (1988) Effects of natural menopause, hysterectomy, and oophorectomy on lumbar spine and femoral neck bone densities. *Obstetrics and Gynecology* **72:** 631–638.

Hudson MM, Greenwald C, Thompson E et al (1993) Efficacy and toxicity of multiagent chemotherapy and low-dose involved-field radiotherapy in children and adolescents with Hodgkin's disease. *Journal of Clinical Oncology* **11:** 100–108.

Jones KP, Ravnikar VA, Tulchinsky D & Schiff I (1985) Comparison of bone density in amenorrheic women due to athletics, weight loss, and premature menopause. *Obstetrics and Gynecology* **66:** 5–8.

Jordan VC, Fritz NF & Tormey DC (1987) Endocrine effects of adjuvant chemotherapy and long-term tamoxifen administration on node-positive patients with breast cancer. *Cancer Research* **47:** 624–630.

Kaufman FR, Loro ML, Azen C et al (1993) Effect of hypogonadism and deficient calcium intake on bone density in patients with galactosemia. *Journal of Pediatrics* **123:** 365–370.

Keilholz U, Korbling M, Fehrentz D et al (1989) Long-term endocrine toxicity of myeloablative treatment followed by autologous bone marrow/blood derived stem cell transplantation in patients with malignant lymphohematopoietic disorders. *Cancer* **64:** 641–645.

Kleczkowska A, Fryns JP & van den Berghe H (1993) Duplication in the long arm of the X-chromosome associated with spastic paraparesis and premature menopause. *Genetic Counseling* **4:** 213–216.

Koyama H, Wada T, Nishizawa Y et al (1977) Cyclophosphamide-induced ovarian failure and its therapeutic significance in patients with breast cancer. *Cancer* **39:** 1403–1409.

Krauss CM, Turksoy RN, Atkins L et al (1987) Familial premature ovarian failure due to an interstitial deletion of the long arm of the X chromosome. *New England Journal of Medicine* **317:** 125–131.

Kreiner D, Droesch K, Navot D et al (1988) Spontaneous and pharmacologically induced remissions in patients with premature ovarian failure. *Obstetrics and Gynecology* **72:** 926–928.

Kreuser ED, Felsenberg D, Behles C et al (1992) Long-term gonadal dysfunction and its impact on bone mineralization in patients following COPP/ABVD chemotherapy for Hodgkin's disease. *Annals of Oncology* **3 (supplement 4):** 105–110.

Kreuser ED, Xiros N, Hetzel WD & Heimpel H (1987) Reproductive and endocrine gonadal capacity in patients treated with COPP chemotherapy for Hodgkin's disease. *Journal of Cancer Research and Clinical Oncology* **113:** 260–266.

Kurabayashi T, Yasuda M, Fujimaki T et al (1993) Effect of hormone replacement therapy on spinal bone mineral density and T lymphocyte subsets in premature ovarian failure and Turner's syndrome. *International Journal of Gynaecology and Obstetrics* **42:** 25–31.

Langevitz P, Klein L, Pras M & Many A (1992) The effect of cyclophosphamide pulses on fertility in patients with lupus nephritis. *American Journal of Reproductive Immunology* **28:** 157–158.

Ledger WL, Thomas EJ, Browning D et al (1989) Suppression of gonadotrophin secretion does not reverse premature ovarian failure. *British Journal of Obstetrics and Gynaecology* **96:** 196–199.

Lonsdale RN, Roberts PF & Trowell JE (1991) Autoimmune oophoritis associated with polycystic ovaries. *Histopathology* **19:** 77–81.

Louis O, Devroey P, Kalender W & Osteaux M (1989) Bone loss in young hypoestrogenic women due to primary ovarian failure: spinal quantitative computed tomography. *Fertility and Sterility* **52:** 227–231.

McDonough PG, Byrd JR, Tho PT & Mahesh VB (1977) Phenotypic and cytogenetic findings in eighty two patients with ovarian failure—changing trends. *Fertility and Sterility* **28:** 638–641.

McNatty KP, Short RV, Barnes EW & Irvine WJ (1975) The cytotoxic effect of serum from patients with Addison's disease and autoimmune ovarian failure on human granulosa cells in culture. *Clinical and Experimental Immunology* **22:** 378–384.

Madsen BL, Giudice L & Donaldson SS (1995) Radiation-induced premature menopause: a misconception. *International Journal of Radiation Oncology, Biology, Physics* **32:** 1461–1464.

Mattison DR, Evans MI, Schwimmer WB, et al., (1984). Familial premature ovarian failure. *American Journal of Human Genetics.* **36:** 1341–1348.

Mehta AE, Matwijiw I, Lyons EA & Faiman C (1992) Noninvasive diagnosis of resistant ovary syndrome by ultrasonography *Fertility and Sterility* **57:** 56–61.

Menon RK, Okonofua FE, Agnew JE et al (1987) Endocrine and metabolic effects of simple hysterectomy. *International Journal of Gynaecology and Obstetrics* **25:** 459–463.

Metka M, Holzer G, Heytmanek G & Huber J (1992) Hypergonadotropic hypogonadic amenorrhea (World Health Organization III) and osteoporosis. *Fertility and Sterility* **57:** 37–41.

Mignot MH, Drexhage HA, Kleingeld M et al (1989) Premature ovarian failure. II: Considerations of cellular immunity defects. *European Journal of Obstetrics, Gynaecology, and Reproductive Biology* **30:** 67–72.

Montz FJ, Wolff AJ & Gambone JC (1991) Gonadal protection and fecundity rates in cyclophosphamide-treated rats. *Cancer Research* **51:** 2124–2126.

Muechler EK, Huang KE & Schenk E (1991) Autoimmunity in premature ovarian failure. *International Journal of Fertility* **36:** 99–103.

Nelson LM, Anasti JN, Kimzey LM et al (1994) Development of luteinized graafian follicles in patients with karyotypically normal spontaneous premature ovarian failure. *Journal of Clinical Endocrinology and Metabolism* **79:** 1470–1475.

Nelson LM, Kimzey LM, White BJ & Merriam GR (1992) Gonadotropin suppression for the treatment of karyotypically normal spontaneous premature ovarian failure: a controlled trial. *Fertility and Sterility* **57:** 50–55.

O'Herlihy C, Pepperell RJ & Evans JH (1980) The significance of FSH elevation in young women with disorders of ovulation. *British Medical Journal* **281:** 1447–1450.

Oldenhave A, Jaszmann, LJ, Everaerd WT & Haspels AA (1993) Hysterectomized women with ovarian conservation report more severe climacteric complaints than do normal climacteric women of similar age. *American Journal of Obstetrics and Gynecology* **168:** 765–771.

Owens S, Roberts WS, Fiorica JV et al (1989) Ovarian management at the time of radical hysterectomy for cancer of the cervix. *Gynecologic Oncology* **35:** 349–351.

Pados G, Camus M, Van Waesberghe L et al (1992) Oocyte and embryo donation: evaluation of 412 consecutive trials. *Human Reproduction* **7:** 1111–1117.

Parker M, Bosscher J, Barnhill D & Park R (1993) Ovarian management during radical hysterectomy in the premenopausal patient. *Obstetrics and Gynecology* **82:** 187–190.

Pellas TC, Ramachandran B, Duncan M et al (1991) Germ-cell deficient (ged), an insertional mutation manifested as infertility in transgenic mice. *Proceedings of the National Academy of Science, USA* **88:** 8787–8791.

Powell CM, Taggart RT, Drumheller TC et al (1994) Molecular and cytogenetic studies of an X;autosome translocation in a patient with premature ovarian failure and review of the literature. *American Journal of Medical Genetics* **52:** 19–26.

Pydyn EF & Ataya KM (1991) Effect of cyclophosphamide on mouse oocyte in vitro fertilization and cleavage: recovery. *Reproductive Toxicology* **5:** 73–78.

Rabinowe SL, Ravnikar VA, Dib SA, et al (1989) Premature menopause: monoclonal antibody defined T lymphocyte abnormalities and antiovarian antibodies *Fertility and Sterility* **51:** 450–454.

Ramahi Ataya AJ, Ataya KM, Subramanian MG & Struck RF (1988) The effect of 'activated' cyclophosphamide on rat granulosa cells in vitro. *Reproductive Toxicology* **2**: 99–103.

Ratcliffe MA, Lanham SA, Reid DM & Dawson AA (1992) Bone mineral density (BMD) in patients with lymphoma: the effects of chemotherapy, intermittent corticosteroids and premature menopause. *Hematological Oncology* **10**: 181–187.

Raymond JP, Izembart M, Marliac V et al (1989) Temporary ovarian failure in thyroid cancer patients after thyroid remnant ablation with radioactive iodine. *Journal of Clinical Endocrinology and Metabolism* **69**: 186–190.

Rebar RW, Erickson GF & Yen SS (1982) Idiopathic premature ovarian failure: clinical and endocrine characteristics. *Fertility and Sterility* **37**: 35–41.

Redman JR, Bajorunas DR, Wong G et al (1988) Bone mineralization in women following successful treatment of Hodgkin's disease. *American Journal of Medicine* **85**: 65–72.

Reichman BS & Green KB (1994) Breast cancer in young women: effect of chemotherapy on ovarian function, fertility, and birth defects. *Monographs of the National Cancer Institute*: 125–129.

Reyno LM, Levine MN, Skingley P et al (1992) Chemotherapy induced amenorrhoea in a randomised trial of adjuvant chemotherapy duration in breast cancer. *European Journal of Cancer* **29A**: 21–23.

Rhim SH, Millar SE, Robey F et al (1992) Autoimmune disease of the ovary induced by a ZP3 peptide from the mouse zona pellucida. *Journal of Clinical Investigation* **89**: 28–35.

Riedel HH, Lehmann Willenbrock E & Semm K (1986) Ovarian failure phenomena after hysterectomy. *Journal of Reproductive Medicine* **31**: 597–600.

Russell P, Bannatyne P, Shearman RP et al (1982) Premature hypergonadotropic ovarian failure: clinicopathological study of 19 cases. *International Journal of Gynecological Pathology* **1**: 185–201.

Samaan NA, deAsis DNJr, Buzdar AU & Blumenschein GR (1978) Pituitary-ovarian function in breast cancer patients on adjuvant chemoimmunotherapy. *Cancer* **41**: 2084–2087.

Sanders JE, Buckner CD, Amos D et al (1988) Ovarian function following marrow transplantation for aplastic anemia or leukemia. *Journal of Clinical Oncology* **6**: 813–818.

Sauer MV, Paulson RJ, Ary BA & Lobo RA (1994) Three hundred cycles of oocyte donation at the University of Southern California: assessing the effect of age and infertility diagnosis on pregnancy and implantation rates. *Journal of Assisted Reproduction Genetics* **11**: 92–96.

Schilsky RL, Sherins RJ, Hubbard SM et al (1981) Long-term follow up of ovarian function in women treated with MOPP chemotherapy for Hodgkin's disease. *American Journal of Medicine* **71**: 552–556.

Sedmak DD, Hart WR & Tubbs RR (1987) Autoimmune oophoritis: a histopathologic study of involved ovaries with immunologic characterization of the mononuclear cell infiltrate. *International Journal of Gynecological Pathology* **6**: 73–81.

Seidenschnur G, Beck H, Uplegger H et al (1989) Attitude and sex behavior following hysterectomy *Zentrablatt für Gynakologie* **111**: 53–59.

Sessums JV & Murphy DP (1932) Hysterectomy and artificial menopause; review of literature, report of 91 cases. *Surgical Gynecology and Obstetrics* **55**: 286–289.

Shalet SM, Beardwell CG, Twomey JA et al (1977) Endocrine function following the treatment of acute leukemia in childhood. *Journal of Pediatrics* **90**: 920–923.

Shalev O, Rahav G & Milwidsky A (1987) Reversible busulfan-induced ovarian failure. *European Journal of Obstetrics, Gynaecology, and Reproductive Biology* **26**: 239–242.

Shiromizu K, Thorgeirsson SS & Mattison DR (1984) Effect of cyclophosphamide on oocyte and follicle number in Sprague-Dawley rats, C57BL/6N and DBA/2N mice. *Pediatric Pharmacology* **4**: 213–221.

Siddle N, Sarrel P & Whitehead M (1987) The effect of hysterectomy on the age at ovarian failure: identification of a subgroup of women with premature loss of ovarian function and literature review. *Fertility and Sterility* **47**: 94–100.

Smith S & Hosid S (1994) Premature ovarian failure associated with autoantibodies to the zona pellucida. *International Journal of Fertility and Menopausal Studies* **39**: 316–319.

Soong YK, Hsu JJ & Tzen KY (1989) Measurement of bone mineral density in amenorrheic women with dual photon absorptiometry. *Taiwan I. Hsueh Hui Tsa Chih* **88**: 1097–1103.

Specht L, Hansen MM & Geisler C (1984) Ovarian function in young women in long-term remission after treatment for Hodgkin's disease stage I or II. *Scandinavian Journal of Haematology* **32**: 265–270.

Spinelli S, Chiodi S, Bacigalupo A et al (1994) Ovarian recovery after total body irradiation and allogeneic bone marrow transplantation: long-term follow up of 79 females. *Bone Marrow Transplant* **14:** 373–380.

Stillman RJ, Schinfeld JS, Schiff I et al (1981) Ovarian failure in long-term survivors of childhood malignancy. *American Journal of Obstetrics and Gynecology* **139:** 62–66.

Strober S, Field E, Hoppe RT et al (1985) Treatment of intractable lupus nephritis with total lymphoid irradiation. *Annals of Internal Medicine* **102:** 450–458.

Tang VW & Faiman C (1983) Premature ovarian failure: a search for circulating factors against gonadotropin receptors. *American Journal of Obstetrics and Gynecology* **146:** 816–821.

Taylor R, Smith NM, Angus B et al (1989) Return of fertility after twelve years of autoimmune ovarian failure. *Clinical Endocrinology.* **31:** 305–308.

Teaff NL, Savoy Moore RT, Subramanian MG & Ataya KM (1990) Vinblastine reduces progesterone and prostaglandin E production by rat granulosa cells in vitro. *Reproductive Toxicology* **4:** 209–213.

Therman E & Susman B (1990) The similarity of phenotypic effects caused by Xp and Xq deletions in the human female: a hypothesis. *Human Genetics* **85:** 175–183.

van Beurden M, Schuster Uitterhoeve AL & Lammes FB (1990) Feasibility of transposition of the ovaries in the surgical and radiotherapeutical treatment of cervical cancer. *European Journal of Surgical Oncology* **16:** 141–146.

van Weissenbruch MM, Hoek A, van Vliet Bleeker I et al (1991) Evidence for existence of a putative role in resistant ovary syndrome? *Journal of Clinical Endocrinology and Metabolism* **73:** 360–367.

Veneman TF, Beverstock GC, Exalto N & Mollevanger P (1991) Premature menopause because of an inherited deletion in the long arm of the X-chromosome. *Fertility and Sterility.* **55:** 631–633.

Waggoner DD, Buist NRM & Donnell GN (1990) Long term prognosis in galactosaemia: results of a survey of 350 cases. *Journal of Inherited Metabolic Disease* **13:** 802–818.

Wallace WH, Shalet SM, Crowne EC et al (1989) Ovarian failure following abdominal irradiation in childhood: natural history and prognosis. *Clinical Oncology of Royal College of Radiologists* **1:** 75–79.

Wallace WH, Shalet SM, Tetlow LJ & Morris Jones PH (1993) Ovarian function following the treatment of childhood acute lymphoblastic leukaemia. *Medical and Pediatric Oncology* **21:** 333–339.

Weetman AP (1995) Autoimmunity to steroid-producing cells and familial polyendocrine autoimmunity. *Baillière's Clinical Endocrinology and Metabolism* **9:** 157–174.

Wheatcroft NJ, Toogood AA, Li TC et al (1994) Detection of antibodies to ovarian antigens in women with premature ovarian failure. *Clinical and Experimental Immunology* **96:** 122–128.

Whitehead E, Shalet SM, Blackledge G et al (1983) The effect of combination chemotherapy on ovarian function in women treated for Hodgkin's disease. *Cancer* **52:** 988–993.

Whitelaw RG (1958) Ovarian activity following hysterectomy. *Journal of Obstetrics and Gynaecology of the British Empire* **65:** 917–932.

Williams RS & Mendenhall N (1992) Laparoscopic oophoropexy for preservation of ovarian function before pelvic node irradiation. *Obstetrics and Gynecology* **80:** 541–543.

Winqvist O, Gebre Medhin G, Gustafsson J et al (1995) Identification of the main gonadal autoantigens in patients with adrenal insufficiency and associated ovarian failure. *Journal of Clinical Endocrinology and Metabolism* **80:** 1717–1723.

Wu RC, Kuo PL, Lin SJ et al (1993) X chromosome mosaicism in patients with recurrent abortion or premature ovarian failure. *Journal of Formos. Medical Association* **92:** 953–956.

3

Psychological and sexual aspects of the menopause and HRT

MARY-JANE PEARCE
KEITH HAWTON

This chapter is about some of the more controversial aspects of the menopause; the nature of the relationship between this time of great hormonal change, psychological disorders, psychiatric illness and disturbance of sexual function, and what effects hormone replacement therapy (HRT) does or does not have on these. There is a high psychological morbidity in all hospital attenders, including those attending the menopause clinic. The problem for the clinician is to identify which, if any, of these psychological symptoms are attributable to the menopause itself, and hence may be responsive to HRT, and when to refer patients back to their GPs for other possible treatments.

Hypotheses of an association between psychological disturbance and reproductive function are longstanding. For example, after Kraeplin described involutional melancholia in 1906, the menopause was for a long time regarded as an aetiological factor in depression. There is now no evidence from research in psychiatry to support this hypothesis. Depression which occurs at this time is not marked by symptoms thought to be characteristic of involutional melancholia (Weissman, 1979). Furthermore, this diagnostic category was abandoned some time ago from both the International Classification of Diseases and Diagnostic and Statistical Manual classification systems.

In the menopause clinic, many women will report enhanced wellbeing following HRT, or may report recurring low mood when it is withdrawn or when an implant is due for replacement. However, research findings have been inconsistent with regard to the response of psychological symptoms to HRT. It may well be that in many women placebo effects are primarily responsible for the responses seen.

Methodological factors in the studies may account for much of the inconsistency (for a review see Pearce et al, 1995), but it is possible to draw some conclusions from the research findings where the most rigorous methodology has been applied.

Baillière's Clinical Obstetrics and Gynaecology—
Vol. 10, No. 3, September 1996
ISBN 0–7020–2177–6
0950–3552/96/030385 + 15 $12.00/00

PSYCHOLOGICAL EFFECTS OF THE MENOPAUSE

There have been many studies associating a range of psychological symptoms with the menopause. However, the prevalence varies depending upon the source from which study populations are drawn. For example, women in clinic samples show more symptoms than do those in general population samples. Surveys of menopause clinic populations (Moore et al, 1975; Garnett et al, 1990) and gynaecology clinic populations (Ballinger, 1975) have indicated very considerable psychological morbidity. For example, 45% of perimenopausal women attending a menopause clinic in Edinburgh were found to be clinically depressed (Hay et al, 1994). But these findings from the menopause clinic may, in part at least, reflect the characteristics of hospital clinic attenders in general, since psychiatric symptoms are frequent in all groups of patients in hospital outpatient settings: estimates of psychiatric cases found among general hospital outpatient populations range from 14 to 52% (Mayou and Hawton, 1986). Furthermore, measures of menopausal symptoms may be affected by other factors such as ageing, physical health status, environmental changes and expectations of the menopause.

A wide variety of psychological symptoms has been found in cross-sectional studies of the menopause. Greene (1984) reviewed 14 cross-sectional general population studies. He concluded that no psychological symptoms followed the same consistent and marked temporal relationship to the menopause as did vasomotor symptoms. While seven studies provided evidence of an increase in psychological symptoms around the time of the menopause, there was little consensus as to which particular symptoms increased and which did not. Moreover, the magnitude of increase was much less than that of vasomotor symptoms and the peak incidence occurred some time prior to the actual menopause.

However, prospective studies provide the best information on psychological symptoms in the menopause since these take account of the women's prior psychological condition. We review these studies in the following section.

Depression and anxiety

Hunter (1990b) prospectively studied psychological and somatic symptoms in a cohort of 36 pre-menopausal women for three years into the peri- or post-menopause. She found a significant, although slight, increase in depressed mood when women became menopausal. When factors contributing to this were examined, psychosocial rather than menopausal ones were significant. For example, current stress and prior hypochondriacal concerns and pre-menopausal negative beliefs about the menopause were found to be implicated.

In the prospective Massachusetts Women's Health Study (MWHS), 2500 pre-menopausal women in the general population were assessed nine-monthly over five years for vasomotor symptoms, menstrual status and depression (McKinlay et al, 1987; Avis et al, 1994). In the MWHS, there was no association between the onset of the natural menopause and risk of depression. However, experiencing a long perimenopause was associated with a transitory increase in depressive symptoms. There was a slight excess of depression in the perimenopause (Avis et al, 1994).

In three other prospective studies, no direct associations between the menopause and depression or psychological wellbeing were found (Matthews et al, 1990; Holte, 1992; Busch et al, 1994). However, Matthews et al (1990) found an increase in depression in the subgroup of women who had become HRT users, while Kaufert et al (1992) found that women who had assessed their physical health as poor pre-menopausally were more likely to become depressed as their menopausal status changed. Similarly, no increase in anxiety was found in three prospective studies in which standardized screening questionnaires were used (Hunter, 1990b; Matthews et al, 1990; Holte, 1992).

Cognitive function

Despite recurrent clinical observations in clinical settings of complaints about the effects of the menopause on memory and concentration, there have been few rigorous studies. In two treatment studies of women immediately following bilateral salpingoophorectomy, mild memory impairments were found at the end of the treatment phase in the women who received placebo rather than oestrogen (Sherwin, 1990; Phillips and Sherwin, 1992).

This is a complex area that requires further investigation since many menopausal women complain of cognitive problems.

Relationship between physical and psychological symptoms

Associations have been found between vasomotor symptoms and psychological symptoms in cross-sectional studies of a gynaecology clinic sample (Ballinger, 1975) and in a general population study of middle-aged women (Gath et al, 1987). Findings from prospective studies are different. Hunter (1990b) found that vasomotor symptoms were not associated with depressed mood state (depressed mood being the only psychological symptom with an association with the menopause in her study). Indeed vasomotor symptoms were predicted by pre-menopausal negative beliefs about the menopause.

However, Holte (1992) found that an increase in social dysfunction was reported after the menopause. Statistical (regression) analysis suggested that this was associated with increased vasomotor complaints.

Non-menopausal factors

Greene (1984a) reviewed seven cross-sectional studies in which social life circumstances and the changes of mid-life were considered. Pre-existing difficulties such as marital dissatisfaction or financial problems were associated with menopausal symptoms, but not events such as children leaving home. This would support a model in which the effects of existing problems are accentuated by the menopause. Greene's own cross-sectional study of a general population sample of women at the climacterium, in which psychosocial factors and reported life events were also measured, has provided some interesting findings (Greene and Cooke, 1980; Cooke and Greene, 1981; Cooke, 1985). The presence and severity of psychological and somatic symptoms was found to be associated directly with life stresses, especially bereavement. In another study, events in mid-life unrelated to the menopause were found to have stronger associations with depression scores than the menopause itself (McKinlay et al, 1987). The strongest associations with depression were found for poor health status, lay health consultation, the use of tranquillizers, and worry about immediate family members (such as adolescent children or ailing parents).

Further evidence of associations between psychosocial factors and depressed mood has come from prospective studies of women passing through the menopause (Hunter, 1990b; Kaufert et al, 1992). It was the women who had initially identified themselves pre-menopausally as under stress who suffered increased rates of depressed mood when they became menopausal. Current minor stresses were also found to be associated with mood disturbance in a prospective study in which the relationships between endocrine status and psychological profiles in HRT users were examined (Alder, 1992).

SEXUAL EFFECTS OF THE MENOPAUSE

There is some lack of clarity in the evidence concerning possible changes in female sexuality with the menopause. While sexual problems are commonly found in women attending gynaecology or specific menopause clinics (Sarrel and Whitehead, 1985), it is in general population studies that the picture is less clear. In part this is because of problems of methodology. In addition to the general methodological problems mentioned above, further problems concern the definition of sexual function and dysfunction. Finally, the male partner's sexuality may influence a woman's sexuality as much as changes within herself (Bachmann et al, 1985), but few studies control for this.

Sexual desire, activity and orgasm

With increasing age, levels of sexual desire (as reflected by self-reports of desire and frequency of sexual fantasies) decrease in both sexes, and low sexual desire becomes more common, particularly in women in their late 40s and 50s (Osborn et al, 1988; Hawton et al, 1994). Similar findings exist with regard to frequency of sexual activity and orgasm. However, it is unclear to what degree the menopause specifically contributes to these changes.

While Pfeiffer and Davies (1972) found that the menopause made only a small statistical contribution to the decline in sexual function, age and marital status being more important, a study by Hallstrom (1977) suggested that menopausal status had a marked effect on sexual interest and on both orgasmic and coital frequency in women aged 45 to 54 years, the effects of age disappearing when the 'climacteric phase' was controlled for. In the UK, Hunter (1990a) found a step-wise decrease in sexual interest across the menopausal stages (pre-, peri- and post-menopausal) which persisted when effects of age were controlled for. A longitudinal study of a small group of women confirmed a decline in sexual desire and coital frequency (but not orgasm) during and following the onset of the menopause, the decline in coital frequency being associated particularly with reduction in serum testosterone levels (McCoy and Davidson, 1985). Cross-sectional studies have found less effect of menopausal status (including specific hormone levels) on sexual function, the effects being some reduction in sexual desire and reduced enjoyment of sexual activity (Bachmann et al, 1985; Hawton et al, 1994).

Thus one can conclude, somewhat tentatively, that reduction in sexual interest, and of frequency of sexual activity with the partner, and, possibly, orgasm, may accompany the menopause. However, this by no means applies to all women, is often not marked, and most women do not develop frank sexual dysfunction at this time. Furthermore, satisfaction with the sexual relationship is unaffected in the majority of women (Hunter, 1990a; Hawton et al, 1994).

Dyspareunia

There is more consistent agreement that dyspareunia frequently accompanies the menopause, together with vaginal dryness. Reduction in vaginal lubrication and vaginal blood flow during sexual stimulation also occur (Leiblum et al, 1983; McCoy and Davidson, 1985). Reduced vaginal lubrication and genital blood flow and engorgement may affect a woman's subjective sense of sexual arousal as well. However, on a more positive note, regular and continued sexual activity appears to protect against vaginal dryness (Leiblum et al, 1983).

Other relevant effects

Changes in mood, wellbeing and self-esteem may all be relevant to sexual adjustment associated with the menopause. In addition, other specific changes may also have a role. For example, changes in general skin sensitivity, including specific complaints about tactile impairment and even unpleasant and painful responses to touch, occur in some post-menopausal women (Sarrel and Whitehead, 1985; Riley, 1989). These effects, which are probably mediated by changes in nerve function resulting from oestrogen deficiency and thinning of the skin, could clearly have sexual consequences. Changes in clitoral sensitivity may also occur. This is usually in the form of reduced sensitivity, which is probably associated with generalized touch impairment (Sarrel and Whitehead, 1985) or decreased clitoral blood flow. Some women, however, experience unpleasant or even painful clitoral hyperaesthesia (Riley, 1991). Either change may interfere with orgasmic capacity. Atrophic changes in the lower urinary tract due to oestrogen deficiency may predispose to greater incidence of the urethral syndrome in post-menopausal women (Brown and Hammond, 1987), a condition exacerbated by sexual intercourse. When this leads to urinary incontinence during sexual activity the consequent embarrassment may interfere with sexual function.

PSYCHOLOGICAL EFFECTS OF HRT

The evidence for the effects of HRT on psychological symptoms associated with the natural menopause is far from clear. Although this aspect of treatment has been examined quite extensively, it is not surprising that findings are unclear given the lack of consensus that an elevation of psychological symptoms is associated specifically with the menopause. As we saw above, depressed mood was the only psychological symptom found to be associated in two of the well-designed prospective studies of women going through the menopause. It is non-menopausal factors that appear to be most relevant when psychological symptoms present.

The evidence for the effects of HRT in treatment studies of oophrectomised women is more consistent.

It may be that methodological problems are obscuring treatment effects. These factors have already been touched upon. In addition, in treatment studies there should be adequate control for the effects of physical symptoms, especially in view of the possible secondary causation of psychological symptoms.

In treatment studies, the double-blind placebo-controlled design will to some extent reduce the bias of non-menopausal factors such as environmental and social changes or expectations of treatment. However, there is considerable variability in the magnitude of placebo effects in this area of research. Placebo effects have been found for both physical and psychological symptoms (Campbell, 1976; Coope, 1976). Several other trials have shown that a placebo preparation can have an effect on vasomotor symptoms as great as that of the active preparation (Strickler et al, 1977; Thomson and Oswald, 1977). However, although the placebo response may be as large as the initial active drug effect, it appears to wane after the first few weeks (Campbell, 1976). Interestingly, Coope (1976) noted that the placebo effect with HRT was only observed in women who received the placebo first in a trial, while those who received the active preparation first reported a return of symptoms during the subsequent placebo phase.

By contrast, a placebo effect has not been found in some trials (Fedor-Freybergh, 1977; Nordin et al, 1981; Brincat et al, 1984; Furuhjelm et al, 1984; Sherwin and Gelfand, 1985; Sherwin et al, 1985; Magos et al, 1986; Sherwin, 1988). Some authors suggest that specific features in the design influence how rigorously blind the study is and will in turn affect the size of the placebo effect: the more rigorous the design the bigger the placebo effect (Coope, 1976; Greene, 1984b).

Effect of oestrogens on psychological symptoms: the natural menopause

There have been a number of treatment trials which were not double-blind in design (Utian, 1972; Schneider et al, 1977; Chakravarti et al, 1979; Durst and Maoz, 1979; Brincat et al, 1984; Cardozo et al, 1984). A range of psychological symptoms was apparently improved and wellbeing was enhanced in these studies.

However, rigorous double-blind treatment studies which used standardized measures of psychological symptoms have produced rather mixed results. From some of these studies there is evidence that, in groups of naturally-menopausal women, oestrogen replacement has positive effects on psychological symptoms and that these are significantly greater than for placebo (Fedor-Freybergh, 1977; Furuhjelm et al, 1984; Montgomery et al, 1987). However, this was not found in other studies (Campbell, 1976; Strickler et al, 1977), where the placebo effects were more marked.

The women in two of these studies suffered from depression; one study suggested that depression improved during HRT (Montgomery et al, 1987) but only in the perimenopausal group, and only at two months after HRT was introduced. There was no difference between placebo and active groups in the post-menopausal women at two months, and no difference for either group at four months. In the second study, HRT had no beneficial effect (Strickler et al, 1977). In a study of severely depressed psychiatric inpatients (Klaiber et al, 1979), a positive effect was found with oestrogens in doses much higher than normally used in HRT; this effect was unrelated to menopausal status.

Two further studies used a double-blind controlled design but non-standardized psychological symptom checklists (Coope, 1976; Gerdes et al, 1982). One of these included a menopausal rating scale as well as a rigorous double-blind control (Coope, 1976). In this study, only hot flushes showed a significant reduction from the active treatment. It is worth drawing attention to the fact that this is one of two studies conducted in a general practice population. The other study, without standardized scales for either menopausal or psychological symptoms, found improvement in complaints of depression and anxiety in women on active treatment (Gerdes et al, 1982).

Effect of oestrogens on psychological symptoms: the surgical menopause

We turn next to prospective treatment studies of HRT in oophrectomized women. Well-controlled studies which used standardized measures of psychological symptoms have more consistently demonstrated improvement in psychological symptoms. For example, Sherwin and Gelfand (1985) studied women with stable relationships and no past or current psychiatric problems (Sherwin and Gelfand, 1985; Sherwin, 1988). In the first study, women were followed prospectively through abdominal hysterectomy and oophorectomy (for benign disease), and those given HRT implants of oestrogen or testosterone were compared with those given placebo (Sherwin and Gelfand, 1985). In the second study, there were two groups of women: those who had been receiving HRT implants for up to four years and a control group of women who had no hormonal treatment during a similar period (Sherwin, 1988). The women who received either of the active implants were found to have a reduction in their depression scores and were also more confident, calm and positive than those who had placebo. In both these studies no reduction in anxiety scores was found. Interestingly, in a further study focused primarily on the effects of oestrogen on cognitive function (see later), Phillips and Sherwin (1992) reported no effect of HRT on measures of anxiety, depression or hostility. Improvement in depression scores was also found in a study by Dennerstein et al (1979). Insomnia and irritability were the most common symptoms to improve with HRT.

In a further study of HRT designed to investigate relationships between endocrine status and psychological profiles in oophorectomized women, Alder (1992) controlled for both vasomotor symptoms and non-menopausal social factors. She demonstrated that minor stresses or 'hassles' contributed more towards the degree of psychological symptoms than did either hormone levels or time since insertion of the implants.

In a recent double-blind placebo-controlled study of 40 women (75% of whom had undergone oophorectomy) who were receiving oestrogen implants at a menopause clinic, half the women who requested a further implant received the oestrogen preparation and the other half received a placebo (Pearce et al, in press). When compared with placebo, receipt of the oestrogen replacement implant did not have significant effects on physical symptoms (except for a non-significant improvement in hot flushes) or psychiatric disorders (in spite of approximately half the women in each group having a psychiatric disorder). In fact, the serum oestradiol levels of nearly all the women were in the pre-menopausal range at the beginning of the study, suggesting that the apparent psychological and other symptoms which led to the women seeking a new implant were mostly unrelated to hormone levels and perhaps more to other factors in their lives.

Effects of oestrogens on cognitive function

Several studies have been conducted in which self-report measures have been used to assess the effects of oestrogens on cognitive function in peri- and post-menopausal women. When objective tests have been used, the results have been variable (Phillips and Sherwin, 1992). This may be because of failure to control for mood or physical symptoms (e.g. hot flushes, sleep disturbance) which are likely to interfere with test perform-ance. In a well-controlled study, Phillips and Sherwin (1992) used a battery of memory tests to study 19 women who, after hysterectomy and oophor-ectomy, had been randomly assigned to receive monthly placebo or oestrogen injections. The design included controls for plasma oestrogen levels, mood and menopausal symptoms. After two months, scores on tests of verbal memory showed a significant decline in the placebo treated group, but not in the oestrogen treated group. No apparent hormonal effects were found on tests of visual memory and attention. The results suggest that specific aspects of memory function may be affected by changes in plasma oestrogen.

Interaction between physical and psychological symptoms

There is evidence from treatment studies to suggest that psychological symptoms may occur secondarily to physical symptoms, especially vasomotor ones (Campbell, 1976; Chakravarti et al, 1979).

Some studies have investigated whether improvements in psychological symptoms occur when physical symptoms improve. An early study which employed non-standardized scales and was only single-blind, described a 'mental tonic' effect (Utian, 1972). That is, oophrectomized women experienced an improvement in psychological wellbeing when physical symptoms improved. However, this was not found in a subsequent study in which mood was assessed using a standardized measure (George et al, 1973).

A 'domino effect' is also described by some authors, whereby improvement in a range of psychological symptoms such as irritability, poor memory, anxiety, worry about age, and insomnia followed alleviation of vasomotor symptoms by oestrogens (Campbell, 1976). In patients without marked physical symptomatology, fewer psychological symptoms significantly improved. A further study found decreases in depression scores associated with alleviation of hot flushes (Dennerstein et al, 1979). There were similar findings in a study by Chakravarti et al (1979) but unfortunately standardized psychological measures were not employed.

By contrast, Furuhjelm et al (1984) found no significant correlation between mental distress scores and vasomotor symptom scores. Thomson and Oswald (1977) studied sleep effects of oestrogen and noted that oestrogen reduced the number of episodes of wakefulness in menopausal women yet made no difference to their anxiety and depression levels.

In summary, it appears that HRT reduces menopausal vasomotor symptoms, although in a minority of controlled studies this effect appeared to be only slightly greater than for placebo. The response of psychological and somatic symptoms is variable and in some studies no greater, or at least not much greater, than for placebo. Placebo effects are variable but probably large when double-blind conditions are rigorous. A 'domino' effect may reasonably describe the improvement in non-vasomotor symptoms after relief from vasomotor symptoms.

Effects of HRT with progestogens and androgens

Norethisterone has been found to reduce hot flushes and sweats but to have no effect on psychological symptoms (Nordin et al, 1981; Paterson, 1982). Magos et al (1986) studied the influence of oral norethisterone on mood and behaviour in a double-blind placebo-controlled study of hysterectomized women receiving testosterone and oestrogen implants for climacteric complaints. Adverse dose-related effects, including negative mood and decreased concentration, were found. Adverse mood effects were also reported when medroxyprogesterone was combined with oestrogen in naturally post-menopausal women (Sherwin, 1991).

Androgens are often given as an adjunct to oestrogen to improve sexual feelings (see below). Sherwin (1988) found that the combination given to oophorectomized women resulted in greater improvement in wellbeing than with oestrogen alone, which was in turn itself more effective than placebo. In contrast, Montgomery et al (1987) did not find greater improvement with adjunct androgen implants. In this study the menopausal HRT users had a high level of psychiatric morbidity. Burger et al (1984) added testosterone to oestrogen therapy in a group of women with persisting menopausal symptoms. This was not a controlled trial, but the women receiving testosterone reported no relief of remaining depression or hot flushes. At present it remains unclear whether androgens have direct benefits on psychological symptoms.

EFFECTS OF HRT ON SEXUAL SYMPTOMS

Sexual desire, arousal and orgasm

Findings have varied between studies with regard to the effects of oestrogen alone on diminished sexual desire associated with the menopause. No effect was found by Utian (1972) who studied oestrogen administration in women who had undergone hysterectomy or oophorectomy, nor by Coope et al (1975) who investigated the effects of oral oestrogen in women presenting for treatment of menopausal symptoms. However, Dennerstein et al (1979) found positive effects of oestrogen treatment on sexual desire, enjoyment and orgasmic frequency (but not on frequency of sexual intercourse) in women who had undergone surgical menopause. Changes in sexual desire and mood were correlated and changes in mood appeared to be partly due to the 'domino effect'. Studies involving progesterone administration alone have found deleterious effects on sexual functioning, including desire and mood (Dennerstein et al, 1979, 1980; Holst et al, 1989).

There is now satisfactory evidence that testosterone supplementation of HRT can have beneficial effects on reduced sexual desire. While Dow et al (1983) and Myers et al (1990) found no advantage of supplementing oestrogen therapy with testosterone for post-menopausal women (natural and surgical) with concerns of reduced sexual interest, other studies have shown convincing evidence of beneficial effects of adding testosterone to the treatment regimen for women whose reduced sexual desire has not responded to oestrogen HRT alone (Cardozo et al, 1984; Burger et al, 1987). In an elegant prospective investigation, Sherwin et al (1985) showed that in surgically menopausal women an oestrogen-androgen combined preparation or androgen alone enhanced the intensity of sexual desire and arousal and frequency of sexual fantasies, whereas little or no such effect was found with either oestrogen alone or placebo. However, actual frequency of sexual intercourse and orgasm were not related to hormone levels.

Vaginal dryness and dyspareunia

There is extensive evidence that oestrogen is usually highly beneficial for the problems of post-menopausal vaginal dryness and dyspareunia, with reversal of atrophic vaginitis (Coope et al, 1975; Campbell, 1976; Brincat et al, 1984).

Other problems

While this review is concerned with HRT for menopausal symptoms, it is important to remember other potential influences on sexuality at this time (e.g. marital adjustment and changes in self-image) and the likelihood that they may merit therapeutic attention in women with sexual complaints.

SUMMARY

Despite the clinical impressions that there are considerable psychological benefits from HRT, there is only clear evidence for amelioration of psychological symptoms (including improvement in cognitive function) in women who have undergone a surgical menopause. Otherwise in the natural menopause it remains unclear which, if any, non-sexual psychological symptoms respond directly to oestrogen except as a secondary response to reduction in physical symptoms. Overall, it has to be said that there is little scientific backing for hormonal treatment of psychological problems on their own around the time of the natural menopause. In most cases psychological treatment or counselling will be more appropriate than HRT.

   It must be remembered that the prevalence of psychological symptoms in the menopause and gynaecology clinic is high just as it is in all hospital settings. The task is to identify which women:

1. Have a predominance of psychological symptoms and might have psychiatric disorders. They may have presented in the clinic because they also happen to be menopausal, but it may well be that the psychiatric disorder has a quite independent aetiology. They will benefit from specific treatment for that disorder.
2. Have, and complain of, low moods or other non-specific psychological symptoms and have presented in the clinic because they are menopausal. They might benefit from practical, supportive help with current and ongoing stresses and strains.
3. Present appropriate menopausal complaints and only on enquiry reveal their psychological problems. In particular, disorders such as depressive illness, anxiety states and alcohol abuse can present with physical

symptoms including ones which mimic vasomotor ones. This group may well be non-responders to HRT.

Women requiring particular consideration might be those with other health problems (particularly chronic ones that might carry on in to old age) who are possibly more at risk of developing depression as they pass through the menopause.

There is clearer evidence that HRT has beneficial effects on sexual function. When sexual symptoms are presented it is worth clarifying the exact features contributing to the complaint. Is it a problem of sexual interest, of infrequency of sexual activity, of vaginal dryness and dyspareunia, or is it a mixture of these complaints?

Reduction of sexual interest and reduced sexual activity with the partner and possibly orgasm may accompany the menopause. Oestrogens have been shown to have some beneficial effect on sexual desire. Where oestrogen alone is ineffective, testosterone is usually beneficial. This treatment effect is particularly clear in surgically menopausal women.

Non-menopausal aspects of the sexual relationship must be considered too. These aspects include the quality of the relationship, the sexual performance of the partner (since sexual desire decreases in both sexes with age), and age-related changes in self-image. These issues may need to be addressed at a simple health education level or with specific counselling. Although a woman's motivation or desire might change as a result of HRT, on its own this will not influence the frequency of intercourse or response during intercourse unless the partner variables permit this.

The situation is more straightforward when problems of post-menopausal vaginal dryness and dyspareunia are the key issues. Oestrogens have been shown to be highly effective in such circumstances. It is also worth noting that regular and continued sexual activity has been found to protect against vaginal dryness.

Acknowledgements

We thank the *British Journal of Psychiatry* for giving permission to use material from our earlier article Pearce et al (1995).

REFERENCES

Alder EM (1992) The effect of hormone replacement therapy on psychological symptoms. In Wijma K and van Schoultz B (eds) *Reproductive Life*. pp 359–362. Carnforth: Parthenon.

Avis NE, Brambilla D, McKinlay SM & Vass K (1994) A longitudinal analysis of the association between menopause and depression. *AEP* **4:** 214–220.

Bachmann GA, Leiblum SR, Sandler B et al (1985) Correlates of sexual desire in post-menopausal women. *Maturitas* **7:** 211–216.

Ballinger CB (1975) Psychiatric morbidity and the menopause: screening of general population sample. *British Medical Journal* **3:** 344–346.

Brincat M, Studd JWW, O'Dowd T et al (1984) Subcutaneous hormone implants for the control of climacteric symptoms: a prospective study. *Lancet* **i:** 16–18.

Brown KH & Hammond CB (1987) Urogenital atrophy. *Obstetrics and Gynaecology Clinics of North America* **15:** 13–32.

Burger HG, Hailes J, Menelaus M et al (1984) The management of persistent menopausal symptoms with oestradiol-testosterone implants: clinical, lipid and hormonal results. *Maturitas* **6**: 351–358.

Burger HG, Hailes J, Nelson J & Menelaus M (1987) Effect of combined implants of oestradiol and testosterone on libido in postmenopausal women. *British Medical Journal* **294**: 936–937.

Busch CM, Zonderman AB & Costa PT (1994) Menopausal transition and psychological distress in a nationally representative sample. *Journal of Aging and Health* **6**: 209–228.

Campbell S (1976) Double blind psychometric studies on the effects of natural oestrogens on post-menopausal women. In Campbell S (ed.) *The Management of the Menopause and Post-Menopausal Years*. pp 149–158. Lancaster: MTP Press.

Cardozo L, Gibb DMF, Tuck SM et al (1984) The effects of subcutaneous hormone implants during the climacteric. *Maturitas* **5**: 177–184.

Chakravarti S, Collins WP, Thom MH & Studd JWW (1979) Relation between plasma hormone profiles, symptoms, and response to oestrogen treatment in women approaching the menopause. *British Medical Journal* **1**: 983–985.

Cooke DJ (1985) Psychosocial vulnerability to life events during the climacteric. *British Journal of Psychiatry* **147**: 71–75.

Cooke DJ & Greene DJ (1981) Types of life events in relation to symptoms at the climacterium. *Journal of Psychosomatic Research* **25**: 5–11.

Coope J (1976) Double blind cross-over study of estrogen replacement therapy. In Campbell S (ed.) *Management of the Menopause and Postmenopausal Years*. pp 159–168. Lancaster: MTP Press.

Coope J, Thomson JM & Poller L (1975) Effects of 'natural oestrogen' replacement therapy on menopausal symptoms and blood clotting. *British Medical Journal* **4**: 139–143.

Dennerstein L, Burrows GD, Hyman GJ & Sharpe K (1979) Hormone therapy and affect. *Maturitas* **1**: 247–259.

Dennerstein L, Burrows GD, Wood C & Hyman G (1980) Hormones and sexuality: effects of oestrogen and progestogen. *Obstetrics and Gynaecology* **51**: 316–322.

Dow MGT, Hart DM & Forrest C (1983) Hormonal treatments of sexual unresponsiveness in post-menopausal women: a comparative study. *British Journal of Obstetrics and Gynaecology* **90**: 361–366.

Durst N & Maoz B (1979) Changes in psychological wellbeing during postmenopause as a result of estrogen therapy. *Maturitas* **1**: 301–315.

Fedor-Freybergh P (1977) The influence of oestrogens on the wellbeing and mental performance in climacteric and postmenopausal women. *Acta Obstetrica et Gynecologica Scandinavica* **(supplement 64)**: 1–91.

Furuhjelm M, Karlgren E & Carlstrom K (1984) The effect of estrogen therapy on somatic and psychical symptoms in postmenopausal women. *Acta Obstetrica et Gynecologica Scandinavica* **63**: 655–661.

Garnett T, Studd JWW, Henderson A et al (1990) Hormone implants and tachyphylaxis. *British Journal of Obstetrics and Gynaecology* **97**: 917–921.

Gath D, Osborn M, Bungay G et al (1987) Psychiatric disorder and gynaecological symptoms in middle aged women. *British Medical Journal* **294**: 213–218.

George GWC, Utian WH, Beaumont PJV & Bearwood CJ (1973) Effects of exogenous oestrogen on minor psychiatric symptoms in postmenopausal women. *South African Medical Journal* **47**: 2387–2388.

Gerdes LC, Sonnendecker EWW & Polakow ES (1982) Psychological changes effected by estrogen-progestogen and clonidine treatment in climacteric women. *American Journal of Obstetrics and Gynecology* **142**: 98–104.

Greene JG (1984a) Symptoms during the climacteric among women in the general population. In: *The Social and Psychological Origins of the Climacteric Syndrome*. pp 40–73. Aldershot: Gower.

Greene JG (1984b) Oestrogen and climacteric symptoms. In: *The Social and Psychological Origins of the Climacteric Syndrome*. pp 12–39. Aldershot: Gower.

Greene JG & Cooke DJ (1980) Life stress and symptoms at the climacterium. *British Journal of Psychiatry* **136**: 486–491.

Hallstrom T (1977) Sexuality in the climacteric. *Clinics in Obstetrics and Gynaecology* **4**: 227–239.

Hawton K, Gath D & Day A (1994) Sexual function in a community sample of middle-aged women with partners: effects of age, marital, socio-economic, psychiatric, gynaecological and menopausal factors. *Archives of Sexual Behavior* **23**: 375–395.

Holst J, Backstrom T, Hammarback S & van Schoultz R (1989) Progestagen addiction during oestrogen replacement therapy: effects on vasomotor symptoms and mood. *Maturitas* **11:** 13–20.

Holte A (1992) Influences of natural menopause on health complaints: a prospective study of healthy Norwegian women. *Maturitas* **14:** 127–141.

Hunter MS (1990a) Emotional well-being, sexual behaviour and hormone replacement therapy. *Maturitas* **12:** 299–314.

Hunter MS (1990b) Somatic experience of the menopause: a prospective study. *Psychosomatic Medicine* **52:** 357–367.

Kaufert PA, Gilbert P & Tate R (1992) The Manitoba Project: a re-examination of the link between menopause and depression. *Maturitas* **14:** 143–155.

Klaiber EL, Broverman DM, Vogel W & Kobayashi Y (1979) Estrogen therapy for severe persistent depressions in women. *Archives of General Psychiatry* **36:** 550–554.

Leiblum S, Bachmann G, Kemmenn E et al (1983) Vaginal atrophy in the post-menopausal woman: the importance of sexual activity and hormones. *Journal of the American Medical Association* **249:** 2195–2198.

McCoy NL & Davidson JM (1985) A longitudinal study of the effects of menopause on sexuality. *Maturitas* **7:** 203–210.

McKinlay JB, McKinlay SJ & Brambilla D (1987) The relative contributions of endocrine changes and social circumstances to depression in mid-aged women. *Journal of Health and Social Behaviour* **28:** 345–363.

Magos AL, Brewster E, Singh R et al (1986) The effects of norethisterone in postmenopausal women on oestrogen replacement therapy: a model for the premenstrual syndrome. *British Journal of Obstetrics and Gynaecology* **93:** 1290–1296.

Matthews KA, Wing RR, Kuller LH et al (1990) Influences of natural menopause on psychological characteristics and symptoms of middle-aged healthy women. *Journal of Consulting and Clinical Psychology* **58:** 345–351.

Mayou R & Hawton K (1986) Psychiatric disorder in the general hospital. *British Journal of Psychiatry* **149:** 172–190.

Montgomery JC, Appleby L, Brincat M et al (1987) Effect of oestrogen and testosterone implants on psychological disorders in the climacteric. *Lancet* **i:** 297–299.

Moore B, Gustafson R & Studd J (1975) Experience of a national health service menopause clinic. *Current Medical Research Opinion* **3 (supplement) 3:** 42–55.

Myers LS, Dixen J, Morrissette D, Carmichael M & Davidson JM (1990) Effects of estrogen, androgen, and progestin on sexual psychophysiology and behavior in postmenopausal women. *Journal of Clinical Endocrinology and Metabolism* 70: 1124–1131.

Nordin BEC, Jones MM, Crilly RG, Marshall DH & Brooke R (1981) A placebo-controlled trial of ethinyl oestradiol and norethisterone in climacteric women. *Maturitas* **2:** 247–251.

Osborn M, Hawton K & Gath D (1988) Sexual function among middle aged women in the community. *British Medical Journal* **296:** 959–962.

Paterson MEL (1982) A randomized double-blind cross-over trial into the effect of norethisterone on climacteric symptoms and biochemical profiles. *British Journal of Obstetrics and Gynaecology* **89:** 464–472.

Pearce J, Hawton K & Blake F (1995) Psychological and sexual symptoms associated with the menopause and the effects of hormone replacement therapy. *British Journal of Psychiatry* **167:** 163–173.

Pearce J, Hawton K & Blake F (in press) Psychological effects of oestrogen implant therapy: a placebo-controlled trial. *Journal of Psychosomatic Research*.

Pfeiffer E & Davies CIC (1972) Determinants of sexual behaviour in middle and old age. *Journal of the American Geriatrics Society* **20:** 151–158.

Phillips SM & Sherwin BB (1992) Effects of oestrogen on memory function in surgically menopausal women. *Psychoneuroendocrinology* **17:** 485–495.

Riley AJ (1989) Post-menopausal touch impairment presenting as sexual avoidance: a case report. *Sexual and Marital Therapy* **4:** 189–194.

Riley AJ (1991) Sexuality and the menopause. *Sexual and Marital Therapy* **6:** 135–146.

Sarrel PM & Whitehead MI (1985) Sex and menopause: defining the issues. *Maturitas* **7:** 217–224.

Schneider MA, Brotherton PL & Hailes J (1977) The effect of exogenous oestrogens on depression in menopausal women. *Medical Journal of Australia* **2:** 162–163.

Sherwin BB (1988) Affective changes with oestrogen and androgen replacement therapy in surgically menopausal women. *Journal of Affective Disorders* **14:** 177–187.

Sherwin BB (1990) Clinical consequences of endocrine changes at the menopause. In van Hall EV and Everaerd W (eds) *The Free Woman: Women's Health in the 1990s.* pp. 680–687. Carnforth: Parthenon.

Sherwin BB (1991) The impact of different doses of estrogen and progestin on mood and sexual behavior in post-menopausal women. *Journal of Clinical Endocrinology and Metabolism* **72:** 336–343.

Sherwin BB & Gelfand MM (1985) Sex steroids and affect in the surgical menopause: a double-blind, cross-over study. *Psychoneuroendocrinology* **10:** 325–335.

Sherwin BB, Gelfand MM & Brender W (1985) Androgen enhances sexual motivation in females: a prospective, crossover study of sex steroid administration in the surgical menopause. *Psychosomatic Medicine* **47:** 339–351.

Strickler RC, Borth R, Cecutti A et al (1977) The role of oestrogen replacement in the climacteric syndrome. *Psychological Medicine* **7:** 631–639.

Thomson J & Oswald I (1977) Effect of oestrogen on the sleep, mood, and anxiety of menopausal women. *British Medical Journal* **ii:** 1317–1319.

Utian WH (1972) The true clinical features of postmenopause and oophorectomy and their response to oestrogen therapy. *South African Medical Journal* **46:** 732–737.

Weissman MM (1979) The myth of involutional melancholia. *Journal of the American Medical Association* **242:** 742–744.

4

Urogenital effects of the menopause

JOSEPH SCHAFFER
J. ANDREW FANTL

The mean age of cessation of menses is 51 years, with an average life expectancy of 27 years beyond that. Women can be expected to live a third of their lives in the post-menopausal state. By the year 2000, there will be 50 million post-menopausal women in the USA (Mishell, 1992). It is therefore expected that management of the gynaecological problems of the menopause will become an increasingly important aspect of routine gynaecological practice (Utian, 1990).

Urogenital disorders are among the most common reasons why menopausal and post-menopausal women seek the aid of a physician (Brown and Hammond, 1987). The menopause occurs at a time when the incidence of degenerative and organic diseases of the urogenital system increases. It is not surprising therefore that associations have been observed between oestrogen deprivation (hypo-oestrogenism) and the urogenital disorders of the menopause. However, scientific evidence supporting many of these associations is lacking. This chapter will discuss the urogenital conditions associated with the menopause and the direct and indirect evidence connecting them to hypo-oestrogenism. Particular emphasis will be placed on the most common syndromes associated with the menopause, including lower genital tract atrophy/atrophic vaginitis, urinary tract infections (UTI) and urinary incontinence. Particular attention will be given to issues of clinical practice.

AGE-RELATED CHANGES OF THE UROGENITAL TRACT

Physiological ageing accelerates at the time of the menopause. On a cellular level, observed changes include: slowing down of cell division and growth, reduced capacity for tissue repair leading to fatty infiltration, cellular atrophy, increased cell pigmentation and degenerative changes in elastic connective tissue. Atrophy of skin and mucosal surfaces occurs along with decreases in skeletal muscle volume and replacement by adipose connective tissue (Brown, 1977). Smooth muscle tone decreases and nerve degeneration occurs.

Baillière's Clinical Obstetrics and Gynaecology—
Vol. 10, No. 3, September 1996
ISBN 0–7020–2177–6
0950–3552/96/030401 + 17 $12.00/00

401

The genital tract

After the menopause, vulvar tissues undergo anatomical and physiological changes. One can observe a loss in vulvar subcutaneous tissue along with a thinning of the epidermis. The labia majora reduce in size and the labia minora may be indistinct. Pubic hair density decreases and the vaginal epithelium becomes less cellular and thinner leading to gradual loss of rugae and obliteration of the fornices. The vagina loses elasticity, shortens, narrows, and becomes less distensible. The decrease in thickness and elasticity allows the vagina to be more readily traumatized and irritated which may lead to bleeding. There is a loss of cellular glycogen which decreases the colonization of Doderlein's bacilli and lactic acid production. As such, vaginal pH increases from approximately 4.0–5.5 to 6.0–8.0 (Utian, 1987). In the post-menopausal alkaline environment, the usual acid pH of the vagina as a potent defence mechanism is lost. This leads to an increased susceptibility to pathogenic bacteria and overgrowth of enteric organisms in the vaginal flora (Klutke and Bergman, 1995). In fact, *Escherichia coli* rarely exists at the introitus when the vaginal pH is <4.5 (Heimer and Englund, 1992). These factors are thought to contribute to the increased prevalence in the elderly of UTI and atrophic vaginitis.

Vaginal atrophy is associated with a decrease in blood flow, a decrease in vaginal fluid and reduced secretion during sexual stimulation and coitus (Semmens and Wagner, 1982; Semmens et al, 1985). In addition, it accounts for 15% of cases of post-menopausal bleeding (Hammond and Maxson, 1982). It is very likely that these physiological changes lead to dyspareunia, a major cause of sexual dysfunction encountered by menopausal women. Thirty-eight per cent of post-menopausal women were found to suffer from vaginal dryness, while 32% lost interest in sex after the menopause (Iosif and Bekassy, 1984).

The lower urinary tract

The genital and urinary tracts develop from a common embryological precursor, the urogenital sinus, therefore the physiological effects of the menopause on the urinary tract are similar to those of the genital tract. The trigonal urothelium thins down as does the epithelium of the urethra. These changes are readily observed in the trigonal areas of squamous epithelium as well as the external urethral meatus. The volume of blood flow through the urethral vascular plexus decreases and pulsations are less evident. These changes lead to a decrease in the normal coaptation of the urethral mucosa. Urethral support may be impaired due to a decrease in the amount and elasticity of the connective tissue supportive structures as well as atrophy of the striated muscle. There is increased cross-linking of collagen and a reduction in the total amount of collagen. Periurethral and urethral α-adrenergic receptors are reduced in number and a gradual slowing of nerve conduction time has been observed. In the bladder, hypertrophy of the detrusor muscle results in an increase in trabeculations and diverticulum. Concomitant loss of the glycosaminoglycan protective layer in the bladder promotes increased susceptibility to bacterial invasion and UTI. In general, the function of the lower urinary tract can be observed to be impaired as bladder capacity decreases. Hypersensitivity of the bladder and urethra increases and the ability to voluntarily suppress or initiate a bladder contraction is reduced (Wall et al, 1993).

Physiological changes associated with ageing in other organ systems affect lower urinary tract function. Impaired cardiac function leads to congestive heart failure, venous stasis, oedema and nocturia. Neurological impairment can lead to decreased awareness of the bladder filling or bladder overactivity. Diabetes may cause increased urine output with associated frequency of urination and nocturia. Peripheral neuropathy in itself may induce both filling and emptying phase dysfunction. Decreased mobility, a consequence of connective tissue ageing can be a major contributor to an altered control over the lower urinary tract.

The prevalence of pelvic organ prolapse increases with age. This occurs due to the cumulative effects of weakening connective tissue, chronic elevation of intra-abdominal pressure, childbirth and genetic predisposition. Pelvic organ prolapse contributes to lower urinary tract dysfunction however, the exact cause and effect are still subjects of debate. Associations include decreased bladder emptying with increased residual urine, urethral sphincter incompetence as well as poorly defined sensory alterations.

HYPO-OESTROGENISM

Oestrogen receptors have been identified in the vagina, cervix, uterus, ovaries, fallopian tubes, urethra, trigone, bladder, connective tissues surrounding the urethra, and the muscles of the pelvic floor (Ingelman-Sundberg, 1981; Brown and Hammond 1987; Rekers et al, 1992). The vagina and urethra, in particular, contain high affinity oestrogen receptors in large concentrations (Iosif et al, 1981; Barbo, 1987). As such, oestrogen plays a major role in the normal maintenance of vaginal and urethral epithelium. These tissues are very susceptible to the decreased levels of circulating oestrogens. Mucosal atrophy has been shown to correlate well with serum oestrogen levels (Capewell et al, 1992; Nilsson and Heimer, 1992a). Women with severe urogenital atrophy had plasma levels of unconjugated oestradiol in the range of 25 to 32 pmol/l with unconjugated oestrone being undetectable (Nilsson and Heimer, 1992a)

The characteristic urogenital changes occurring during the menopause are due to the combination of physiological ageing and hypo-oestrogenism, but the exact contribution of each of these is difficult to ascertain and is likely to vary between individuals. During the menopause, oestrogen is derived mostly from peripheral (adipose tissue) aromatization of androstenedione to oestrone and conversion of oestrone to oestradiol; therefore the amount of circulating oestrogen depends to an extent on the amount of body fat. As an example of individual variability, urogenital atrophy develops shortly after cessation of menses in some women and years later or never in others.

Lower genital tract atrophy

Prevalence and symptoms

While the exact prevalence of symptomatic lower genital tract atrophy is unknown, clinical experience would suggest that it is common. Many women with vaginal atrophy are relatively free of symptoms while others suffer from pain, burning, dryness, discharge, dyspareunia, decreased vaginal lubrication and vaginal bleeding. These symptoms are among the most common reasons why menopausal and post-menopausal women seek health care. A survey study in Sweden looked at the prevalence of genito-urinary symptoms in women of 61 years of age (Iosif and Bekassy, 1984). It was found that 15% of post-menopausal women complained of vaginal itching, discharge and pain, 38% suffered from vaginal dryness and dyspareunia and 32% had lost interest in sexual relations. Another survey study by Rekers et al (1992) showed that 10% of post-menopausal women suffered from vaginal pain, 23% itching, 22% discharge and 16% dyspareunia.

In a study of sexual dysfunction in menopausal women, Sarrel (1990) noted a direct correlation between oestradiol levels below 50 pg/ml and symptoms of vaginal dryness, dyspareunia and burning. The individual response to low levels of circulating oestrogen varies widely. Atrophic changes tend to occur later than other oestrogen-related menopausal symptoms because relatively less oestrogen is necessary to maintain the vaginal epithelium. However, a decrease in vaginal lubrication may be one of the first symptoms of hypo-oestrogenism even in pre-menopausal women (Beard, 1992).

Diagnosis

Urogenital atrophy is often subjectively assessed by visually evaluating the appearance of the vaginal mucosa. Clinically, atrophy is thought to be present if the vaginal epithelium is thin, pale and dry, without rugae and the introital size is reduced. An objective assessment of atrophy can be made by obtaining a vaginal smear from the upper lateral third of the vagina. An oestrogen-deficient smear is one in which parabasal cells are dominant and superficial cells are minimal. Several numerical indices have been proposed which attempt to assess oestrogenic activity. Among these are the Karyopyknotic Index and the Maturation Index. The Karyopyknotic Index measures the relationship of superficial cells to intermediate cells regardless of cytoplasmic staining. The Maturation Index represents the percentile of superficial, intermediate and parabasal cells (Blaustein, 1987). Because oestrogen stimulates maturation of the vaginal epithelium from the basal to the superficial level, in general a post-menopausal vaginal smear tends to progress from a decrease in superficial cells to a complete absence. The presence of parabasal cells shed from the deep epithelial layer suggests atrophy. The cytological picture can vary considerably, and in some women an oestrogenic effect on the vaginal epithelium may be present for years after the menopause (Notelovitz, 1978). In one study of women over 75 years of age, 25% showed some superficial cells on cytological smear (McLennan and McLennan, 1971).

Capewell et al (1992) attempted to correlate subjective assessment of atrophy with the cytological smear. Moderate or severe atrophy on smear occurred in 90% of patients with symptoms of vaginal dryness. The other physical signs commonly associated with atrophy (mucosal pallor, dryness, petechiae, lack of pubic hair and reduced introital size) did not correlate with the degree of atrophy determined by cytology. This suggests that a combination of subjective (symptoms) and objective (cytology) evaluation will improve diagnostic accuracy.

Treatment

Lower genital tract atrophy responds to oestrogen administration. Different types of oestrogen are used as well as different routes of administration. The therapeutic effect may depend on the type of oestrogen, the dose, the vehicle and the route of administration (Baker, 1994).

Three separate classes of oestrogen are used for oestrogen replacement therapy. These include natural oestrogens: oestradiol, oestrone and oestriol, conjugated equine oestrogens (CEO), and synthetic oestrogens: ethinyl oestradiol, quinesterol and diethylstilbesterol (Lobo, 1987). Each of these oestrogens has been used to treat lower genital tract atrophy through either the vaginal, oral, transdermal or subcutaneous routes.

While oral oestrogen has been effective for the treatment of atrophy, vaginal administration is often chosen because it avoids the enterohepatic circulation and exerts a rapid local effect. Oestrogen can be administered vaginally as a cream, tablet or slow release from a vaginal ring or pessary. Creams are currently available containing CEO, 17β-oestradiol, estropipate, dienestrol and oestriol. CEO contains 0.625 mg of conjugated oestrogens in each gram of cream. Although the manufacturer of CEO recommends cyclic administration of 0.5 to 2 g daily, in actuality, several different dosing schemes have been used.

Mandel et al (1983) studied the effects of vaginal CEO on the vaginal epithelium and found that a daily dosage of 0.3 mg for four weeks returned vaginal cytology to the pre-menopausal range. The effect of 0.3 mg on the vaginal epithelium was similar to that exerted with 1.25 mg of oral CEO. This suggests that on a per milligram basis, the potency of vaginal CEO is fourfold greater than that of oral CEO on the vaginal epithelium. In a similar study, Dyer et al (1982) treated 24 menopausal patients with atrophy using 0.1, 0.4, 0.8 or 1.25 mg of CEO cream nightly for a month. Vaginal smears were obtained to assess epithelial cell proliferation and maturation. After one week vaginal cytology was in the pre-menopausal range in the patients of each group. The maximal response was at two weeks, after which values declined but still remained within the pre-menopausal range, suggesting a progressive loss of epithelial sensitivity to oestrogen. While higher doses of CEO may be necessary to relieve vasomotor symptoms, this study showed that low doses relieve atrophy. It is suggested that failure to obtain symptomatic relief be treated not by increasing the dose but by stopping treatment for a short period and then restarting at a lower dose. Handa et al (1994) treated patients with 0.3 mg of vaginal CEO daily for two weeks and then three times per week for six months. Symptoms were relieved and all had significant improvement in vaginal cellular maturation. The correct dosage of vaginal CEO may vary per individual, however, it would be prudent to follow the manufacturer's recommendation and choose the lowest dose that controls symptoms.

The duration of therapy with vaginal CEO necessary to reverse and prevent future atrophy is unknown. In Dyer's study, only patients receiving the lowest dose, 0.1 mg, maintained vaginal cytology in the pre-meno-pausal range four weeks after discontinuing therapy (Dyer et al, 1982).

Oestradiol is also used in the treatment of vaginal atrophy as a cream, transdermally, or tablet and vaginal ring form. Nilsson and Heimer, (1994) treated 10 women with severe urogenital atrophy with low-dose trans-dermal administration of 12.5 µg daily (Estraderm TTS) of 17β-oestradiol twice weekly. After four weeks of treatment, there was a significant decrease in parabasal cells and an increase in intermediate and superficial cells. The gynaecological examination showed less vaginal atrophy after treatment and subjectively there was an improvement in symptoms of dryness and soreness.

Vaginal tablets containing 17β oestradiol are also used for treating atrophy (Mettler and Olsen, 1991; Eriksen and Rasmussen, 1992; Nilsson and Heimer, 1992b). In one study, women were treated with vaginal tablets containing 25 µg of 17β-oestradiol daily for two weeks followed by a twice-weekly maintenance dose for 10 weeks. After three months of therapy, vaginal cytology showed a disappearance of parabasal cells and there was clinical and subjective improvement in symptoms.

Vaginal rings containing 17β oestradiol are currently being used as a vehicle for hormone replacement therapy (HRT). These rings are placed in the upper third of the vagina and release a constant dose of oestradiol for up to three months. Doses as low as 6.5 µg daily have been found effective in reversing atrophy and relieving symptoms (Holmgren et al, 1989; Mattsson et al, 1989; Smith, 1993; Henriksson et al, 1996). Vaginal creams containing 17β oestradiol (Estrace) and oestriol are also commonly used worldwide and have been found to be effective in the treatment of atrophy.

While vaginal administration of oestrogen is an effective treatment for vaginal atrophy it has the potential to produce systemic effects. Absorption of oestrogen by the vaginal epithelium is extremely efficient though it depends on the vehicle through which the oestrogen is delivered; if oestrogen is suspended in saline, absorption is rapid with very high serum levels of oestrogen within one hour. After administering 0.5 mg of 17β-oestradiol in saline vaginally, Schiff et al (1977) found a 29-fold increase in serum oestradiol at one hour. At six hours, the mean plasma oestradiol level was still eightfold higher than pre-treatment levels. When delivered as a vaginal cream, Mandel et al (1983) showed that serum levels of oestrogens are approximately 25% of those achieved with a comparable oral dose, thus the cream vehicle appears to retard vaginal absorption.

Of concern are the possible effects of unopposed vaginal oestrogen on the endometrium. A MEDLINE literature search failed to identify any cases of endometrial carcinoma resulting from vaginal oestrogen use, yet there have been several reports of endometrial proliferation and hyperplasia with vaginal oestrogen therapy (Luisi et al, 1980). However, these studies used high-dose vaginal oestrogen (>3 mg) and not all had pre-treatment endometrial biopsies. In a study by Handa et al (1994), 20 patients with documented atrophic endometrium were treated with 0.3 mg vaginal CEO for six months. One patient developed endometrial hyperplasia. The American College of Obstetricians and Gynecologists (1992) technical bulletin recommends concomitant use of progestogen therapy for women receiving vaginal oestrogen. Although the risk of developing endometrial carcinoma is very low, a prudent strategy would be to cyclically withdraw patients with progestogen therapy. Should bleeding occur after periodic withdrawal, a further evaluation for endometrial proliferation would need to be initiated.

Alternatives to oestrogen

Unfortunately, not all women with urogenital atrophy are candidates for oestrogen supplementation. Several alternative therapies have been proposed including Tamoxifen, water-based jellies, creams and oils, vegetable oil, polycarbophil and yogurt. At the present time, there is limited data regarding the effectiveness of these treatments (Miller, 1992). Retrospective data exist to suggest that continued sexual activity may prevent the development of vaginal atrophy by maintaining epithelial blood flow and pH in the normal range (Leiblum et al, 1983).

Conclusion

Low-dose vaginal oestrogen therapy effectively treats lower genital tract atrophy. Other routes of administration are also effective but the smaller dose required with the vaginal route and the decreased systemic absorption make it the preferred choice. The vehicle of delivery (cream, tablet, ring) does not seem to affect the success of treatment. Likewise, each of the types of oestrogens described provide effective therapy. Should therapy not be successful, it may be discontinued and restarted a few weeks later. The appropriate duration of therapy is unknown. Because there is potential for systemic absorption and endometrial proliferation, concomitant progestogen therapy should be considered in all patients receiving vaginal oestrogen.

THE LOWER URINARY TRACT AND THE MENOPAUSE

Post-menopausal women suffer from an increasing incidence of disorders of the lower urinary tract. Recurrent UTI and urinary incontinence will be discussed.

Recurrent UTI

The prevalence of symptomatic and asymptomatic UTI increases with age (Karafin and Coll, 1987; Heimer and Englund, 1992). Studies have shown an increase in the prevalence of UTI in women beginning in their mid 50s increasing from 5% in a group from 45 to 54 years of age, to 10% in women from 55 to 64 years of age, to 15% in women older than 65 years (Privette et al, 1988). The aetiology of this increase is hypothesized to be due to several factors: hypo-oestrogenism leads to atrophic mucosal changes of the vagina, urethra and bladder resulting in increased vaginal pH, altered vaginal flora and increased bacterial colonization with unfavourable flora such as *E. coli* (Orlander et al 1992; Raz and Stamm 1993). The loss of the glycosaminoglycan protective layer in the bladder may also lead to increased susceptibility to bacterial invasion (Wall et al, 1993). Other factors include increased post-void residuals, impaired bladder emptying, increased faecal and urinary incontinence, and the increased incidence of bladder trabeculations and diverticula.

Symptoms

Symptoms of UTI include frequency, urgency, dysuria, haematuria and incontinence. However, the presence of these symptoms does not always reliably predict infection (Staskin, 1986). Thirty to 40% of patients suspected of having UTI based on symptoms will have sterile urine (Orlander et al, 1992). Therefore, the diagnosis should always be confirmed by either urinalysis or urine culture. If these are negative, work-up for other causes of the patient's symptoms should be initiated. In addition, in the menopause, urinary infections do not always present with the standard symptoms of cystitis and therefore urine culture should be considered a part of the standard evaluation of fever of unknown origin, flank pain and incontinence.

Treatment

Chronic suppressive antibiotic therapy is frequently employed in the management of recurrent UTI in the elderly. While this may be successful in sterilizing the urine, it does not treat the underlying condition. Oestrogen therapy has been proposed as a prophylactic treatment for recurrent UTI in the post-menopausal woman with urogenital atrophy. Several uncontrolled studies have attempted to treat elderly women with recurrent UTIs with prophylactic vaginal oestrogen therapy. Parsons and Schmidt (1982) treated five post-menopausal women with severe recurrent cystitis with intra-vaginal oestrogen. At entry, all the patients were colonized with entero-bacter and had an elevated vaginal pH >5.2. After oestrogen therapy, all the patients returned to a normal vaginal pH and had disappearance of bacterial pathogens. Remaining on low-dose intravaginal oestrogen, four out of the five patients had no further evidence of infection. In another uncontrolled study, 12 women with an average of 3.9 UTI a year were treated with oral or vaginal oestrogen (Privette et al, 1988). The incidence of UTI in this group decreased from 83 in 24 months to four in 24 months. In a randomized, double-blind trial, Raz and Stamm (1993) treated post-menopausal women with recurrent UTI with intravaginal oestriol cream 0.5 mg nightly for two weeks and then twice a week for eight months. In the treated group, the mean vaginal pH declined from 5.5 to 3.8, the rate of vaginal colonization with Enterobacteriaceae fell from 67 to 31% and there was a significant reduction in the incidence of UTIs. While these results are provocative, they remain unconfirmed and other studies have come to differing conclusions (Orlander et al, 1992).

Because there is strong evidence that oestrogen therapy reverses mucosal atrophy, decreases vaginal pH and decreases colonization with bacterial pathogens all potential risk factors for recurrent UTI, it would seem prudent to consider a trial of intravaginal oestrogen in post-menopausal women who suffer from atrophy and recurrent UTIs. It should also be kept in mind however, that asymptomatic bacteriuria is common in post-menopausal women and most authorities do not recommend antibiotic treatment as it leads to development of resistant organisms (Baldessarre and Kaye, 1991).

Urinary incontinence and lower urinary tract dysfunction

The majority of studies on the epidemiology of urinary incontinence indicate that the prevalence increases with age (Teasdale et al 1988; Molander et al, 1990; Milsom et al 1993). Several factors may be responsible for this increase, including the decrease in oestrogen occurring after the menopause. However, hypo-oestrogenism as an independent factor within the ageing process has not been scientifically proven to induce urinary incontinence by itself.

Prevalence rates vary depending on definitions, study design, population and geographical location. In the USA, a survey study revealed that in non-institutionalized women over 60 years of age, 37.7% suffered from incontinence (Diokno et al, 1986). In a population of institutionalized elderly patients with a mean age of 87 years, 41% were found to be incontinent (Resnick et al, 1989). In a review of prior studies, Herzog and Fultz (1990) found the prevalence to range from 8 to 34% among older persons. In the same study the prevalence of severe incontinence, defined as at least a weekly episode or more, was 3 to 11%. In addition, it was noted that 33% of all geriatric incontinence may be transient. While incontinence is more common in the old than the young, approximately two-thirds of elderly women do not suffer from incontinence and thus it should not be considered a normal part of ageing.

Numerous epidemiological studies have looked at incontinence through the life cycle and attempted to correlate the onset of incontinence with the menopause. In a survey study of 902 Swedish women 61 years of age, 29% complained of incontinence and 70% of these related the onset of these symptoms to the menopause. (Iosif and Bekassy, 1984) In a random sample of 1746 Swedish women from 40 to 66 years of age, 10% had 'troublesome' incontinence but there was no difference in the rates of peri- and post-menopausal incontinence (Hagstad and Janson 1986). Osborne (1976) interviewed 600 working women from 35 to 60 years of age and was unable to show an increase in the prevalence of stress incontinence at the time of the menopause. Thomas et al (1980) surveyed 10 000 women and was also unable to show a rise in the prevalence of regular incontinence at the time of the menopause. It is therefore likely that the menopause per se does not represent a precipitating factor although ageing and/or hypo-oestrogenism may be either a co-aetiological factor or may aggravate a previously present condition.

Versi et al (1995) evaluated 324 women who had never had HRT who were attending a menopause clinic in England. There did not appear to be any change in the prevalence of incontinence in the first five years after the menopause. Some of the specific symptoms such as stress urinary incontinence began to decline five years after the menopause. This decline in incontinence after the middle of the fifth decade was also observed by Jolleys (1988). The prevalence of urge incontinence did not change with time from the menopause however, frequency of urination and nocturia increased. Pain on micturition was reported by 10% of patients but there was no trend in the prevalence of this symptom with advancing age. Urodynamic studies did not reveal statistically significant trends with respect to age from the menopause. Using videourodynamic testing, Versi (1990) found no difference in the rate of bladder neck incompetence between peri- and post-menopausal women, suggesting that the integrity of the urethral sphincter may not be oestrogen-dependent. His work provides some support to the hypothesis that some forms of incontinence and voiding difficulties are not directly exacerbated by oestrogen deprivation.

While it is not surprising that the symptom of incontinence has been clinically and temporally associated with the menopause, epidemiological and observational studies do not provide conclusive evidence that the overall prevalence of incontinence relates directly either to the menopause or to hypo-oestrogenism.

The lower urinary tract

Anatomy and physiology

The function of the lower urinary tract is the storage and evacuation of urine. For normal function to occur the bladder must fill with urine with minimal increases in intravesical (detrusor) pressure. This process, unique to the bladder, is known as accommodation. During the storage phase, bladder sensation should also be negligible such that one is not usually aware of the bladder filling. Bladder capacity must also be within a normal range for normal storage to occur and the reservoir function to be maintained. The urethral sphincter functions as a closed valve maintaining urine within the bladder until the appropriate time and place for evacuation. During the storage phase the urethral sphincter must maintain a pressure (resistance) higher than intravesical pressure and withstand sudden increases in intra-abdominal and intravesical pressure. Disorders of the storage phase lead to symptoms of urgency, frequency and urinary incontinence.

The evacuation phase depends on the ability to voluntarily initiate and sustain a detrusor contraction coincident with a relaxation of the urethral sphincter. Disorders of the evacuation phase induce inadequate voiding which may lead to increased post-void residual volume, decompensated detrusor function and upper urinary tract decompensation.

In women, the entire urethra represents the urethral sphincter. It is composed of mucosa, a vascular bed, connective tissue, and smooth and striated muscle fibres. Urethral pressure or resistance is derived from each of these anatomical components although the exact contribution of each component in the elderly is not known (Fantl et al, 1994).

Both the bladder and urethral sphincter are under the control of the central and peripheral nervous systems. The autonomic nervous system has both parasympathetic and sympathetic representation. The parasympathetic system predominates over the bladder while the sympathetic predominates over the urethral sphincter particularly through α-adrenergic receptors located in the bladder neck. The central nervous system, in the form of a complex series of reflex arcs involving autonomic and somatic nerves, modulates bladder and urethral function. The co-ordination of these reflexes allows for efficient filling and emptying. It is the maturation of the central and peripheral nervous system reflex arcs in childhood which allows for successful toilet training and acquisition of continence. Prior to this maturation, emptying occurs spontaneously, without volitional control, when the bladder fills to a critical volume.

Pathophysiology

It has been suggested that the lower urinary tract, as in other organ systems, has a normal physiological level of function and a reserve function. This reserve function is put to work when physiology is impaired (Fantl, 1994). Lower urinary tract changes as previously noted occur as women age. These changes demand compensatory mechanisms to preserve the continence status which, if not adequate, may precipitate the onset of incontinence. It is therefore hypothesized that the elderly lack the necessary reserve that younger women have and thus similar precipitating factors (drug effects, exertion etc.) may alter the continence status.

Figure 1 is a schematic representation of continence and incontinence (the storage phase). Factors affecting the storage phase are specifically listed in Table 1. Most of these are thought to be affected by ageing although the exact mechanisms are not known.

Types and mechanisms of urinary incontinence

Genuine stress incontinence and detrusor instability are the most common types of urinary incontinence in post-menopausal women. Genuine stress incontinence represents the leakage of urine occurring during increases in intra-abdominal pressure and is thought to be due to an inadequate

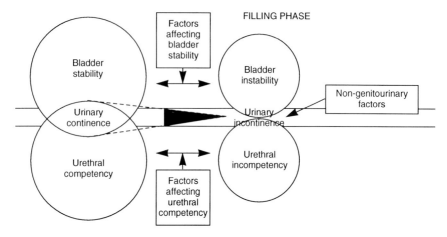

Figure 1. Lower urinary tract function. Reproduced from Fantl (1994, *Experimental Gerontology* **29:** 417–422 © Elsevier Science Inc) with permission.

Table 1. Factors contributing or resulting in urinary incontinence.

Genitourinary factors
  Affecting detrusor stability
    CNS control
    PNS integrity and function
    Bladder wall distensibility
    Intrinsic stimulation
    Extrinsic stimulation

  Affecting urethral sphincteric function

Passive:	**Dynamic:**
Mucosa	Physical exertion
Striated muscle	Urethral axial mobility
Smooth muscle	Vesical pressure
Collagen fibres	Pressure transmission
Elastic fibres	Voluntary striated muscle contraction
Vascular plexus	Reflex striated muscle contraction

Non-genitourinary factors
  Cognitive function
  Psychological function
  Functional ability
  Environmental issues

Reproduced from Fantl (1994, *Experimental Gerontology* **29:** 417–422 © Elsevier Science Inc) with permission.

sphincter mechanism. The aetiology of the inadequate sphincter is thought to be multifactorial however, two major subgroups have been identified; patients whose sphincteric mechanism is defective because of hyper-mobility of the urethra but whose sphincteric function is otherwise normal, and patients whose condition is due to inadequate intrinsic sphincter function. Hypermobility of the urethral axis is considered a major factor in the pathophysiology of genuine stress incontinence, particularly in young women. In such cases, the sphincter mechanism of the urethra is intact but its mobility during exertion impairs the transmission of pressure to the sphincter and predisposes to leakage. Atrophy seems to reduce urethral mobility in older women, however impaired transmission may be seen in these patients. Other factors such as decreased periurethral tissue elasticity and density may be the reason for the observed decrease in pressure transmission during exertion. In addition, neuromuscular denervation, mucosal atrophy and muscular deterioration may represent added conditions leading to genuine stress incontinence in older persons.

Detrusor instability represents a type of incontinence due to involuntary contractions of the bladder which cannot be suppressed. This condition is most frequently thought to be idiopathic, with more than 90% of women having no recognizable aetiology (Karram, 1993). There are several conditions of the central and peripheral nervous system which can cause detrusor instability. These include cerebrovascular accidents, tumours, Parkinson's disease and diabetes. Other conditions such as pelvic organ prolapse and chronic UTI may also lead to detrusor instability. All these diseases or conditions increase with age and therefore may be the epidemiological determinant of the increased prevalence of urge incontinence in the elderly.

The normal function of the lower urinary tract and the continence mechanism is based on anatomy, physiology and learned behaviour. A reserve function is likely to exist and be used to overcome insufficiencies determined by either disease, trauma, or the ageing process. Failure to compensate for the insufficiencies may result in urinary incontinence or other lower urinary tract syndromes. Most of our knowledge of how ageing and the menopause affect continence is lacking, and both basic and clinical research is needed to elucidate these issues. Without an understanding of the ageing process effect on the function of the lower urinary tract, therapeutic trials will remain poorly focused.

ROLE OF OESTROGEN

While the sensitivity of the bladder and urethra to oestrogens has long been recognized, its specific role in the aetiology, pathogenesis and treatment of lower urinary tract dysfunctions is poorly understood.

Semmelink et al (1990) observed abrupt age-independent decreases in smooth muscle tissue in the lamina propria of the trigone and proximal urethra, as well as in the superficial muscular layer of the vagina, trigone and urethra, in women at the time of the menopause. These observations suggest a hormonally-related phenomenon. He also found that young ovariectomized women had the same histological appearance of the lower urogenital tract. In addition, hormonally-induced smooth muscle atrophy of the lower urinary tract was so characteristic that women could be classified as pre- or post-menopausal accordingly. Decreased urethral pressure after the menopause may be due to lack of oestrogens or to age-dependent changes such as decreased circulation, insufficient stimulation of α-adrenergic receptors, and atrophy of soft tissue (Semmelink et al 1990).

This study supports hormonally-induced age-independent smooth muscle atrophy as a cause of reduced urethral pressure.

Several attempts have been made to test the theory that incontinence is related specifically to hypo-oestrogenism. In a double-blind study, Walter et al (1978) looked at the effect of oestrogen on urinary incontinence in post-menopausal women. Patients received oestradiol 2 mg or oestriol 1 mg for four months. Subjectively, oestrogen was superior to placebo in curing frequency, urgency and urge incontinence. Of the 21 patients with these symptoms, eight were cured subjectively, only one of whom got a placebo. There was, however, no change in symptoms of stress incontinence. Two other double-blind placebo-controlled trials of oestrogen therapy (Samsioe et al, 1985; Eriksen and Rasmussen, 1992) showed significant improvement in urge incontinence but a larger trial by Cardozo et al (1993) failed to do so.

In a retrospective study, Fantl et al (1988) compared clinical and urodynamic variables in 23 oestrogen- and 49 non-oestrogen-supplemented post-menopausal women with urinary incontinence. No direct effect of oestrogen supplementation was noted on parameters of urethral function. In patients with detrusor instability, a borderline effect was noted in the volume needed to reach maximum cystometric capacity from the first sensation to void. Nocturia was significantly less frequent in the oestrogen-supplemented group. This led to the hypothesis that a possible beneficial effect of oestrogen in post-menopausal women was an increase in the proprioceptive sensory threshold of the bladder. Other evidence in the study which supports a sensory modulating effect of oestrogen is decreased nocturia, a higher presence of positive bulbocavernosus reflex and a lower prevalence of symptoms of urge incontinence in the oestrogen-supplemented subjects. Previous investigators have also shown that irritative symptoms in post-menopausal women, with or without incontinence, seem to respond to oestrogen supplementation.

A meta-analysis published in 1994 reviewed much of the world literature relating to the efficacy of oestrogen therapy in the treatment of post-menopausal urinary incontinence (Fantl et al, 1994). Of 166 studies, only 23 met quality criteria. Of those subjected to meta-analysis, six were controlled trials and 17 were an uncontrolled series. A subjective improvement in incontinence was found, but the data do not provide strong evidence of an effect of oestrogen therapy on urodynamic variables or objective outcome. This study pointed out that there is a disappointing lack of scientific evidence supporting the independent use of oestrogen in the treatment of post-menopausal urinary incontinence.

A recent unpublished randomized, placebo-controlled, double-blinded trial looked at the efficacy of cyclic HRT on urinary incontinence in hypo-oestrogenic women. The women were treated for three months with oral conjugated oestrogens (0.625 mg) and cyclic oral medroxyprogesterone. Outcomes evaluated were the number of incontinent episodes per week, fluid loss, voluntary diurnal and nocturnal micturitions, and quality of life questionnaires. No significant difference in any outcome variable was found between the placebo and oestrogen group (Fantl, in press).

Conclusion

Oestrogen receptors have been identified in the tissues of the urethra, bladder and pelvic floor musculature. Sensitivity and responsiveness to oestrogens has been noted in epithelial, connective, muscle and vascular tissues. Urodynamic testing has observed that variations in oestrogen influence urethral vascular pulsations, urethral closure pressure and urethral pressure transmission. These reports, in addition to the epidemiological data related to the prevalence of lower urinary tract dysfunction after the menopause have led to the hypothesis that hypo-oestrogenism is a factor in the development of urinary incontinence and that oestrogen replacement therapy might represent an effective treatment. Review of the literature does not support this hypothesis. It is likely that hypo-oestrogenism is one of several factors involved in the ageing process and while it may contribute to the development of incontinence, it is not a singular causative factor. Oestrogen supplementation as an adjunct to other therapies such as medications, behavioural modification, or surgery may prove to be of benefit.

REFERENCES

American College of Obstetricians and Gynecologists (1992) Hormone replacement therapy. *ACOG Technical Bulletin* **166:** Washington, DC.

Baker VL (1994) Alternatives to oral estrogen replacement: Transdermal patches, percutaneous gels, vaginal creams and rings, implants, and other methods of delivery. *Obstetrics and Gynecology Clinics of North America* **21(2):** 271–297.

Baldassarre JS & Kaye D (1991) Special problems of urinary tract infection in the elderly. *Medical Clinics of North America* **75(2):** 375–390.

Barbo DM (1987) The physiology of the menopause. *Medical Clinics of North America* **71(1):** 11–19.

Beard MK (1992) Atrophic vaginitis. *Postgraduate Medicine* **91(6):** 257–260.

Blaustein RL (1987) Cytology of the female genital tract. In Kurman RJ (ed.) *Blaustein's Pathology of the Female Genital Tract.* pp 876–898. New York: Springer-Verlag.

Brown ADG (1977) Postmenopausal unary problems. *Clinics in Obstetrics and Gynaecology* **4(1):** 181–206.

Brown KH & Hammond CB (1987) Urogenital atrophy. *Obstetrics and Gynecology Clinics of North America* **14(1):** 13–32.

Capewell AE, McIntyre MA & Elton RA (1992) Post-menopausal atrophy in elderly women: Is a vaginal smear necessary for diagnosis? *Age and Aging* **21:** 117–120.

Cardozo L, Rekers H, Tapp A et al (1993) Oestriol in the treatment of postmenopausal urgency: A multicentre study. *Maturitas* **18:** 47–53.

Diokno AC, Brock BM, Brown MB & Herzog AR (1986) Prevalence of urinary incontinence and other urological symptoms in the noninstituionalized elderly. *Journal of Urology* **136:** 1022–1025.

Dyer GI, Young O, Townsend PT et al (1982) Dose-related changes in vaginal cytology after topical conjugated equine oestrogens. *British Medical Journal* **284:** 789.

Eriksen PS & Rasmussen H (1992) Low-dose 17 beta-estradiol vaginal tablets in the treatment of atrophic vaginitis: A double-blind placebo controlled study. *European Journal of Obstetrics, Gynecology and Reproductive Biology* **44(2):** 137–144.

Fantl JA (1994) The lower urinary tract in women–effect of aging and menopause on continence. *Experimental Gerontology* **29:** 417–422.

Fantl JA, Bump RC, Robinson D et al (1996) Efficacy of estrogen supplementation in the treatment of urinary incontinence. *Obstetrics & Gynecology* (in press).

Fantl JA, Cardozo L & McClish DK (1994) Estrogen therapy in the management of urinary incontinence in postmenopausal women: A meta-analysis. First report of the hormones and Urogenital Therapy Committee. *Obstetrics and Gynecology* **83:** 12–18.

Fantl JA, Wyman JF, Anderson RL et al (1988) Postmenopausal urinary incontinence: Comparison between non-estrogen-supplemented and estrogen-supplemented women. *Obstetrics and Gynecology* **71(6):** 823–828.

Hagstad A & Janson PO (1986) The epidemiology of climacteric symptoms. *Acta Obstetrica et Gynecologica Scandinavica* **134 (supplement):** 59.

Hammond CB & Maxson WS (1982) Current status of estrogen therapy for the menopause. *Fertility and Sterility* **37(1):** 5–24.

Handa VL, Bachus KE, Johnston WW et al (1994) Vaginal administration of low-dose conjugated estrogens: Systemic absorption and effects on the endometrium. *Obstetrics and Gynecology* **84(2):** 215–218

Heimer GM & Englund DE (1992) Effects of vaginally-administered oestriol on post-menopausal urogenital disorders: A cytohormonal study. *Maturitas* **14:** 171–179.

Henriksson L, Stjernquist M, Boquist L et al (1996) A one-year study of efficacy and safety of a continuous, low-dose, estradiol-releasing ring (Estring) in postmenopausal women with symptoms and signs of urogenital aging. *American Journal of Obstetrics and Gynecology* **174(1):** 85–92.

Herzog AR & Fultz NH (1990) Prevalence and incidence of urinary incontinence in community-dwelling populations. *Journal of the American Geriatrics Society* **38:** 273–281.

Holmgren PA, Lindskog M & von Schoultz B (1989) Vaginal rings for continuous low-dose release of oestradiol in the treatment of urogenital atrophy. *Maturitas* **11:** 55–63.

Ingelman-Sundberg A, Rosen J, Gustafsson SA & Carlstrom K (1981) Cytosol estrogen receptors in the urogenital tissues in stress-incontinent women. *Acta Obstetrica et Gynecologica Scandinavica* **60:** 585–586.

Iosif CS, Batra S & Ek A (1981) Estrogen receptors in the human female lower urinary tract. *American Journal of Obstetrics and Gynecology* **141:** 817.

Iosif CS & Bekassy L (1984) Prevalence of genito-urinary symptoms in the late menopause. *Acta Obstetrica et Gynecologica Scandinavica* **63:** 257–260.

Jolleys JV (1988) Reported prevalence of urinary incontinence in women in a general practice. *British Medical Journal* **296:** 1300–1302.

Karafin LJ & Coll ME (1987) Lower urinary tract disorders in postmenopausal woman. *Medical Clinics of North America* **71(1):** 111–121.

Karram MM (1993) Detrusor instability and hyperreflexia. In Walters MD and Karram MM (eds) *Clinical Urogynecology.* pp 264. St Louis: Mosby.

Klutke JJ & Bergman A (1995) Hormonal influence on the urinary tract. *Urologic Clinics of North America* **22(3):** 629–639.

Leiblum S, Bachman G, Kemmann E et al (1983) Vaginal atrophy in the postmenopausal woman. *Journal of the American Medical Association* **249:** 2195.

Lobo RA (1987) Absorption and metabolic effects of different types of estrogens and progestogens. *Obstetrics and Gynecology Clinics of North America* **14(1):** 143–167.

Luisi M, Franchi F & Kicovic PM (1980) A group-comparative study of effects of ovestrin cream versus premarin cream in post-menopausal women with vaginal astrophy. *Maturitas* **2(4):** 311–319.

McLennan MT & McLennan CE (1971) Estrogenic status of menstruating and menopausal women assessed by cervicovaginal smears. *Obstetrics and Gynecology* **37:** 325.

Mandel FP, Geola FL, Meldrum DR et al (1983) Biological effects of various doses of vaginally administered conjugated equine estrogens in postmenopausal women. *Journal of Clinical Endocrinology and Metabolism* **57(1):** 133–139.

Mattsson LA, Cullberg G, Eriksson O & Knutsson F (1989) Vaginal administration of low-dose estradiol—effects on the endometrium and vaginal cytology. *Maturitas* **11:** 217–222.

Mettler L & Olsen PG (1991) Long-term treatment of atrophic vaginitis with low-dose oestradiol vaginal tablets. *Maturitas* **14(1):** 23–31.

Miller KL (1992) Alternatives to estrogen for menopausal symptoms. *Clinical Obstetrics and Gynecology* **35(4):** 884–893.

Mishell DR (1992) Menopause. In Herbst AL, Mishell DR, Stenchever MA and Droegemueller W (eds) *Comprehensive Gynecology* pp. 1245. St Louis: CV Mosby.

Milsom I, Ekelund P, Molander U et al (1993) The influence of age, parity, oral contraception, hysterectomy and menopause on the prevalence of urinary incontinence in women. *Journal of Urology* **149:** 1459–1462.

Molander U, Milsom I, Ekelund P & Mellstrom D (1990) An epidemiological study of urinary incontinence and related urogenital symptoms in elderly women. *Maturitas* **12:** 51–60.

Nilsson K & Heimer G (1992a) Endogenous estrogen levels in postmenopausal women with severe urogenital atrophy. *Gynecology Obstetrics Investigation* **34**: 234–236.

Nilsson K & Heimer G (1992b) Low-dose estradiol in the treatment of urogenital oestrogen deficiency—a pharmacokinetic and pharmacodynamic study. *Maturitas* **15**: 121–127.

Nilsson K & Heimer G (1994) Ultra-low-dose transdermal estrogen therapy in postmenopausal urogenital estrogen deficiency—a placebo-controlled study. *Menopause: The Journal of the North American Menopause Society* **1(4)**: 191–197.

Notelovitz M (1978) Gynecologic problems of menopausal women: Part 1. Changes in genital tissue. *Geriatrics* **33(8)**: 24–30.

Orlander JD, Jick SS, Dean AD & Jick H (1992) Urinary tract infections and estrogen use in older women. *Journal of the American Geriatrics Society* **40**: 817–820.

Osborne JL (1976) Postmenopausal changes in micturition habits and in urine flow and urethral pressure studies. In Campbell S (ed.) *The Management of the Menopause and Postmenopausal Years*. MTP Publications.

Parsons CL & Schmidt JD (1982) Control of recurrent lower urinary tract infection in the postmenopausal woman. *Journal of Urology* **128(6)**: 1224–1226.

Privette M, Cade R, Peterson J & Mars D (1988) Prevention of recurrent urinary tract infections in postmenopausal women. *Nephron* **50**: 24–27.

Raz R & Stamm WE (1993) A controlled trial of intravaginal estriol in postmenopausal women with recurrent urinary tract infections. *New England Journal of Medicine* **329(11)**: 753–756.

Rekers H, Drogendijk AC, Valkenburg HA & Riphagen F (1992) The menopause, urinary incontinence and other symptoms of the genito-urinary tract. *Maturitas* **15**: 101–111.

Resnick NM, Yalla SV & Laurino E (1989) The pathophysiology of urinary incontinence among institutionalized elderly persons. *New England Journal of Medicine* **320(1)**: 1–7.

Samsioe G, Jansson I, Mellstrom D & Svanborg A (1985) Occurrence, nature and treatment of urinary incontinence in a 70-year-old female population, *Maturitas* **7**: 335–342.

Sarrel PM (1990) Sexuality and menopause. *Obstetrics and Gynecology* **75** (**supplement 4**): 26S–30S.

Schiff I, Tulchinsky D & Ryan KJ (1977) Vaginal absorption of estrone and 17β-estradiol. *Fertility and Sterility* **28(10)**: 1063–1066.

Semmelink HJF, de Wilde PCM, van Houwelingen JC & Vooijs GP (1990) Histomorphometric study of the lower urogenital tract in pre- and post-menopausal women. *Cytometry* **11**: 700–707.

Semmens JP & Wagner G (1982) Estrogen deprivation and vaginal function in postmenopausal women. *Journal of the American Medical Association* **248(4)**: 445–448.

Semmens JP, Tsai CC, Semmens EC & Loadholt CB (1985) Effects of estrogen therapy on vaginal physiology during menopause. *Obstetrics and Gynecology* **66(1)**: 15–18.

Smith P (1993) Estrogens and the urogenital tract. *Acta Obstetrica et Gynecologica Scandinavica* **72** (**supplement 157**): 5–26.

Staskin DR (1986) Age-related physiologic and pathologic changes affecting lower urinary tract function. *Clinics in Geriatric Medicine* **2(4)**: 701–709.

Teasdale TA, Taffet GE, Luchi RJ & Adam E (1988) Urinary incontinence in a community-residing elderly population. *Journal of the American Geriatrics Society* **36**: 600–606.

Thomas TM, Plymat KR, Blannin J & Meade TW (1980) Prevalence of urinary incontinence. *British Medical Journal* **281**: 1243.

Utian WH (1987) The fate of the untreated menopause. *Obstetrics and Gynecology Clinics of North America* **14(1)**: 1–11.

Utian WH (1990) Current perspectives in the management of the menopausal and postmenopausal patient: Introduction. *Obstetrics and Gynecology* **75** (**supplement 4**): 1S–2S.

Versi E (1990) Incontinence in the climacteric. *Clinical Obstetrics and Gynecology* **33(2)**: 392–398.

Versi E, Cardozo L, Studd J et al (1995) Urinary disorders and the menopause. *Menopause: The Journal of the North American Menopause Society* **2(2)**: 89–95.

Wall LL, Norton PA & DeLancey JOL (1993) Special considerations in the elderly. In *Practical Urogynecology* pp. 316–331. Baltimore: Williams & Wilkins.

Walter S, Wolf H, Barlebo J & Jensen HK (1978) Urinary incontinence in postmenopausal women treated with estrogens. *Urology International* **33**: 135–143.

5

The uterus and the menopause

MARGARET C. P. REES

On average, women will experience 400 menstruations between the menarche and the menopause. Endometrial development during the menstrual cycle is ultimately under the hormonal control of oestradiol and progesterone, and will continue to respond in the post-menopause to replacement steroids. This chapter will examine the process of endometrial growth and the mechanisms of endometrial bleeding; and the amount of bleeding with the effect on compliance. Treatment options in terms of bleeding patterns and safety will be discussed. The final section will explore methods of endometrial assessment.

ENDOMETRIAL GROWTH AND MECHANISMS OF ENDOMETRIAL BLEEDING

Endometrial development during each menstrual cycle involves extensive angiogenesis. Regeneration of the microvasculature is initiated from remaining post-menstrual arteriolar stumps in the basalis and includes well differentiated coiled arterioles, capillaries and venules (Kaiserman-Abramof and Padykula, 1989). Neither oestrogen nor progesterone has intrinsic angiogenic activity. Endometrial angiogenesis must be mediated indirectly since steroid receptors are present on endometrial glandular epithelium and stroma but not on endothelium (Perrot-Applanat et al, 1988). Known angiogenic polypeptides include acidic and basic fibroblast growth factors (aFGF and bFGF), vascular endothelial growth factor (VEGF) and the related placental growth factor (PLGF), transforming growth factor $\beta1$ (TGF-$\beta1$), pleiotropin for which there is a related gene midkine (MK) and the platelet derived endothelial cell growth factor (PDECGF) now known to be thymidine phosphorylase (Zhang et al, 1995). Regulators of angiogenesis whose expression has been identified either in whole endometrium or isolated endometrial epithelium and stroma in culture are FGF, VEGF, TGF-$\beta1$, pleiotropin (PT) and MK (Zhang et al, 1995). The only mRNA not detected was PLGF. It is interesting that for decidual/endometrial endothelial growth in vitro only VEGF stimulates

Baillière's Clinical Obstetrics and Gynaecology—
Vol. 10, No. 3, September 1996
ISBN 0–7020–2177–6
0950–3552/96/030419 + 14 $12.00/00

419

growth, suggesting an important role for this angiogenic regulator (Grimwood et al, 1995). While expression of mRNA for both VEGF and MK by isolated normal endometrial epithelial cells shows a twofold increase, that of TGF-β1 decreases fourfold on treatment with a physiological dose of 17β-oestradiol. Furthermore, expression of TGF-β1 is abolished by exposure to progesterone. It is likely that the steroids used in hormone replacement therapy (HRT) act on the endometrium in a similar manner. One study has found changes in bFGF expression in the endometrium of women taking HRT, with levels similar to pre-menopausal endometrium (Rusnati et al, 1993).

The process of menstruation is restricted to humans and certain subhuman primates such as rhesus monkeys. The role of the endometrial vasculature in menstruation was provided by Markee's (1940) remarkable experiments in rhesus monkeys in which he transplanted pieces of endometrium to the anterior chamber of the eye where they became attached and became vascularized. Such explants bled into the aqueous humor at the time of menstruation and responded to hormonal stimulation and deprivation as did the endometrium at its normal site. He estimated that the majority of blood that is lost during menstruation is from endometrial spiral arterioles, rather than capillaries and venules (Markee, 1940). The principal candidates controlling endometrial haemostasis are prostaglandins and fibrinolytic proteins (Rees, 1989), but data regarding these agents under the influence of HRT are limited. During menstruation, these arterioles undergo profound vasoconstriction with bleeding occurring as they dilate, and it is probable that the same process occurs during withdrawal bleeds induced by HRT.

With regard to the ultrastructure of endothelium exposed to cyclical monthly HRT, arterioles are poorly developed and the lumen of the vessels reduced by somewhat hypertrophic immature, endothelial cells which contain a large nucleus and little densely packed cytoplasm. In specimens collected at the onset of the withdrawal bleed, gaps are evident between vacuolated endothelial cells with breaks in the basement membrane allowing migration of erythrocytes into the surrounding stroma (Rees and Sheppard, 1993) (Figure 1).

BLEEDING AND COMPLIANCE

Bleeding is one of the most important issues in continuing HRT (Coope and Marsh, 1992; Barentsen et al, 1993; Hope and Rees, 1995). In Britain, only 15% of women aged between 45 and 54 years take HRT (National Opinion Poll 1994) and most only take it for a few months which denies long-term benefit, a situation which is found in many other countries. A recent survey of British women showed that the main intolerable side effect of HRT was heavy bleeding. Thus it is important to increase the treatment options in terms of bleeding patterns, especially for women well past the menopause who wish no bleed or infrequent bleed regimens.

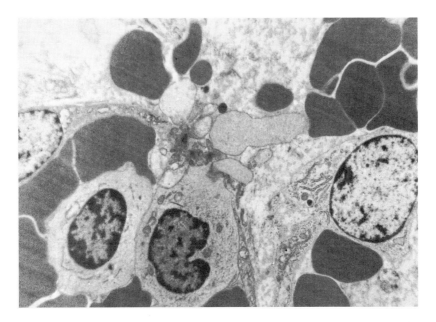

Figure 1. Ultrastructure of an endometrial arteriole during a withdrawal bleed showing a break in the endothelium.

Treatment options

The treatment options are monthly sequential oestrogen–progestogen regimens which result in monthly bleeds in most women, long cycle HRT and so-called 'no bleed' HRT. Monthly sequential and long cycle HRT are suitable for both peri- and post-menopausal women. 'No bleed' HRT is only suitable for post-menopausal women. If given in peri-menopausal women, it results in unacceptable irregular bleeding (Udoff et al, 1995).

BLEEDING PATTERNS WITH HRT

How much blood is lost with HRT?

Most women using sequential oestrogen-progestogen HRT will experience regular withdrawal bleeds. Blood loss has been quantified with monthly cyclical HRT, but as yet there are no data with long cycle HRT. Objective measurement is essential since women are poor judges of their menstrual loss (Fraser et al, 1984). Blood loss can easily be measured using the alkaline haematin technique (Hallberg and Nilsson, 1964). In a normal pre-menopausal population, median blood loss is 35 ml and the 90th percentile is 80 ml (Hallberg et al, 1966). Blood loss has been examined on various preparations. In one study, the combination of 2 mg oestradiol valerate for 21 days with either 250 µg levonorgestrel or 10 mg medroxyprogesterone acetate for the last 10 days for three months in 29 women was examined. Here median blood loss for the levonorgestrel and medroxyprogesterone acetate was 22 (range, 0–582) and 15.6 ml (range, 0–346), respectively (Sporrong et al, 1992). In another study, 50 women given oestradiol valerate 2 mg daily continuously with levonorgestrel 75 μg for the last 12 days of each 28-day cycle, were followed-up for one year (Rees and Barlow, 1991). Two women did not bleed throughout the study. In the remainder, median blood losses were 26 ml at three months (range, 1–313), 23 ml at six months (range, 2–256) and 17 ml at 12 months (range, 1–106). Thus, withdrawal bleeds induced by monthly cyclical HRT are similar to those found in a normal pre-menopausal population, but are greater than those in women taking the combined oral contraceptive pill (Cole et al, 1971).

Duration of bleeding

The average duration of menstrual bleeding is five to six days ($n = 321$) (Rees, unpublished observations (Figure 2)). With monthly sequential regimens, mean duration varies between three and seven days (Rees and Barlow, 1991; Sporrong et al, 1992; Archer et al, 1994). There was no difference in duration when different doses of progestogen were compared (5 and 10 mg medroxyprogesterone acetate) (Archer et al, 1994). With long cycle HRT, inducing bleeds every three months, duration varies form five to seven days (Ettinger et al, 1994; Williams et al, 1994; Hirvonen et al 1995).

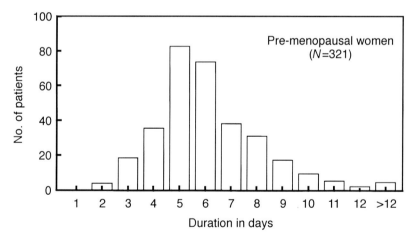

Figure 2. Duration of menstruation in 321 pre-menopausal women (Rees, unpublished observations).

How to achieve amenorrhoea

To avoid bleeding, and thus increase compliance, continuous combined oestrogen-progestogen regimens have been advocated. These were first introduced in a large series by Staland (1981). The rationale regarding the mode of action of continuous combined regimens, is that the continuous progestogen stimulation will keep the endometrium atrophic. This has been shown in long-term use in women treated for a mean of 3.9 years, where the endometrium was examined both hysteroscopically and histologically (Hawthorn et al, 1991). It is not unusual for women to bleed during the first six months of therapy, and in most cases it is light bleeding or spotting. The frequency of bleeding decreases over time and at 12 months most women are amenorrhoeic (Christiansen and Riis, 1990). The incidence of bleeding is lower the longer the woman has been post-menopausal (Staland, 1981; Archer et al, 1994). Irregular bleeding is more frequent if continuous combined regimens are used in perimenopausal women, and therefore such regimens should be reserved for post-menopausal women who have experienced their last period at least six months previously. The same proviso applies to tibolone, a compound with combined oestrogenic, progestogenic and androgenic actions; but here 12 months' amenorrhoea is recommended before starting treatment.

However, some perimenopausal women, especially those with menor-rhagia, wish to have an amenorrhoeic regimen on HRT. Population studies have reported that the amount of blood loss in women around 50 years of age is larger than that of younger women (Hallberg et al, 1966). Amenorrhoea cannot be reliably achieved with oral delivery of the progestogen because of the high incidence of irregular bleeding. Uterine delivery of the progestogen levonorgestrel in an intrauterine contraceptive device results in amenorrhoea and is an effective treatment for menor-rhagia. This device has been used in 18 perimenopausal women with the oestrogen administered orally. After 12 months' treatment, 15 of the women were amenorrhoeic and endometrial biopsies showed no sign of prolifer-ation (Andersson et al, 1992). The oestrogen can also be delivered by other routes such as oestradiol implants (Suhonen et al, 1995).

Other no bleed regimens have been suggested; using interrupted progestogen, using alternating cycles of three days with and without progestogen, or giving the progestogen for five days a week (Mishell et al, 1991; Casper and Chapdelaine, 1993).

LONG CYCLE HRT

The concept of long cycle HRT was introduced to reduce the frequency of withdrawal bleeds in perimenopausal women, and to increase the options for post-menopausal women who find continuous combined HRT un-suitable. Three-monthly, four-monthly and even six-monthly regimens have been described (David et al, 1993; Ettinger et al, 1994; Lafferty and Fiske, 1994; Williams et al, 1994, Hirvonen et al 1995). Three-monthly regimens induce bleeding similar to pre-menopausal periods and are described below in further detail. One series examined four-monthly regimens: here 528 women were treated with 17β-oestradiol 2 mg/day followed by norethisterone 1 mg/day for 10 days in addition to oestradiol in the fourth cycle for six years. While simple endometrial hyperplasia was seen in the third cycle, this had disappeared after the fourth cycle (David et al, 1993). Six-monthly regimens have also been described, but there are few endometrial data (Kemp et al, 1989; Lafferty and Fiske, 1994).

Endometrial safety

Endometrial safety is of prime importance in women taking HRT. The main concern is that the preparation should not induce endometrial malignancy or a pre-malignant hyperplasia. Endometrial cancer is not common in the general population, with approximately 3% of 50-year-old women developing the disease over the remainder of their lives (Grady et al, 1995).

There have been several classifications of hyperplasia over the years. In reality, the only important distinction, in both prognostic and therapeutic terms, between the various forms of hyperplasia is between those which are associated with a significant risk of evolving into an endometrial adeno-carcinoma and those devoid of any such risk. It is now generally agreed that the defining and only feature of an endometrial hyperplasia which is indicative of a potentiality for malignant change is cytological atypia (Fox and Buckly, 1982). Hence the fundamental subdivision of endometrial hyperplasia is into those with cytological atypia and those lacking this feature. Thus hyperplasias can be classified into those with:

1. Cytological atypia, classed as atypical hyperplasia.
2. Without cytological atypia; subdivided into simple and complex forms, the latter having architectural atypia where the risk of progression to malignant disease is less than 5% over 13 years (Kurman et al, 1985).

In 1975, the link between unopposed post-menopausal oestrogen replacement therapy and endometrial cancer was established (Smith et al, 1975). Not long after, the addition of progestogen was found to reduce the risk of endometrial hyperplasia and carcinoma (Gambrell, 1978; Gambrell et al, 1980). The effect of unopposed oestrogen therapy increasing the risk of developing endometrial hyperplasia and carcinoma has recently been reviewed in a meta-analysis of 30 studies (Grady et al, 1995). The summary relative risk (RR) was 2.3 for oestrogen users compared to non-users with a 95% confidence interval (CI) of 2.1–2.5. The relative risk increased with prolonged duration of use (RR 9.5 for 10 or more years). The summary RR of endometrial cancer remained elevated for five or more years after discontinuation of unopposed oestrogen therapy (RR 2.3). Interrupting oestrogen from five to seven days per month was not associated with a lower risk than daily use. Users of unopposed conjugated oestrogen had a greater RR of developing endometrial cancer than users of synthetic oestrogens. The risk of endometrial cancer death was also elevated in un-opposed oestrogen users (RR 2.7, CI 0.9–8.0).

The addition of progestogen has been advocated for many years with the intention of preventing hyperplasia and carcinoma. Ten days or more of progestogen therapy are recommended for monthly sequential regimens (Paterson et al, 1980). Meta-analysis of oestrogen-progestogen HRT shows that the overall summary RR for endometrial cancer was 0.8 (CI 0.6–1.2), but the direction of the effect was different in cohort versus case control studies; 0.4 (CI 0.2–0.6) and 1.8 (CI 1.1–3.1), respectively (Grady et al, 1995). Cohort studies are generally considered to be methodologically superior to case-control studies, mainly because the potential for recall bias in the latter design is avoided. It should be noted however, that the cohort studies analysed included only 10 cases of endometrial cancer (Hammond et al, 1979; Gambrell et al, 1980; Persson et al 1989). Two studies provide information on the effect of the number of days per month that progestogen was used with oestrogen. In the study by Voigt et al (1991), women who took progestogen for fewer than 10 days per month had an RR for endometrial cancer of 2.0 compared to 0.9 for those who took progestogen for at least 10 days per month. In contrast, in the case-control study by Brinton and Hoover (1993), the RR for endometrial cancer was 1.8 and did not vary for the number of days per month that progestogen was used. Further studies are clearly needed to examine the effect of oestrogen-progestogen regimens on endometrial cancer.

The response to progestogen can be assessed in several ways. In addition to endometrial histology, endometrial histochemical markers such as oestradiol and isocitrate dedydrogenase, serum placental protein 14, or markers of endometrial proliferation such as Ki67 can be used (Byrjalsen et al, 1992; Darj et al, 1995).

The level of protection that should be achieved by an individual oestrogen-progestogen combination needs to be addressed. Should the aim be for a zero hyperplasia rate or one that is similar to that found in post-menopausal women not taking HRT? The former is unrealistic and probably unachievable. In a study of 801 perimenopausal and post-menopausal women with no abnormal bleeding, before enrollment into a multicentre study of oestrogen-progestogen replacement, 41 (5.2%) were found to have endometrial hyperplasia, four had atypical hyperplasia and one had an endometrial cancer (Archer et al, 1991). This yield is less than that of Koss et al (1984), who found 16 cases of endometrial carcinoma in 2586 women on first screening at a rate of 6.2 per 1000. However, this group is not comparable to that of Archer et al (1991), since 21.8% were oestrogen users and were solicited for the purpose of cancer screening resulting in self-selection bias which may have increased the risk in this population. In fact, Koss et al (1984) believed that some women concealed symptoms of abnormal bleeding.

In a recent study of 413 women taking monthly sequential HRT, complex hyperplasia was found in 11 (2.7%) (Sturdee et al, 1994). No atypical hyperplasia was reported. Similar rates of simple or complex hyperplasia have been found with three-monthly regimens (Ettinger et al, 1994; Hirvonen et al, 1995). Continuous combined therapy has been examined in a recent meta-analysis of 42 studies published since 1981 (Udoff et al, 1995). Almost all studies, regardless of the hormonal preparations used, reported endometrial atrophy rates of 90 to 100%, even after only three months of treatment. With regard to endometrial hyperplasia, the largest study to date (533 women) by Woodruff et al (1994) found that after one year of treatment, the combined continuous regimen of conjugated equine oestrogen 0.625 mg/day with medroxyprogesterone acetate either 2.5 or 5 mg/day produced a rate of endometrial hyperplasia of less than 1%. No atypical endometrial hyperplasia was reported. Notable exceptions to these findings are the two cases of endometrial adenocarcinoma reported by Leather et al (1991); however both these women had, at one time during therapy, an endometrial biopsy revealing atypical endometrial hyperplasia. It could be argued that given the malignant potential of atypical hyperplasia, they should not have been administered any HRT, but treated surgically.

ENDOMETRIAL ASSESSMENT

Endometrial assessment is a much vexed question with regard to its appropriate use and the technique employed, which the following section will attempt to answer.

When should the endometrium be assessed?

There is no need to assess the endometrium routinely before starting HRT in women with no abnormal bleeding. Abnormal bleeding consists of a sudden change in menstrual pattern, intermenstrual bleeding, post-coital bleeding or a post-menopausal bleed. Here endometrial assessment is essential before starting HRT.

When taking HRT again, women with abnormal bleeding need to be assessed. On cyclical HRT, abnormal bleeding is denoted by a change in pattern of withdrawal bleeds and breakthrough bleeding. Until recently, the evidence suggested that the pattern of withdrawal bleeding was a guide to endometrial histology; a bleed starting on or after day 11 of the progestogen phase was thought to give reassurance of a normal endometrium (Padwick et al, 1986). However, a more recent study in a larger number of women suggests that 2.7% of women with appropriately timed withdrawal bleeds have complex hyperplasia (Sturdee et al, 1994). There is often concern if women do not have a withdrawal bleed on cyclical HRT. However, this simply reflects an atrophic endometrium and does not warrant investigation, except in women with a premature menopause where pregnancy has to be excluded.

In women taking a continuous combined regimen, bleeding may occur at the start of treatment but usually stops after a few weeks; if it persists for more than four to six months, or is not lessening, endometrial assessment is required. Similarly, women who are amenorrhoeic on a continuous combined regimen and then have a bleed need to be assessed.

Why should the endometrium be assessed?

Endometrial assessment is undertaken to detect endometrial abnormalities. The ones of concern are endometrial hyperplasias, polyps and carcinoma. It must be remembered that endometrial adenocarcinoma is rare under 45 years of age.

METHODS OF ASSESSMENT

The main methods of assessment are endometrial biopsy, hysteroscopy, and vaginal ultrasound.

Endometrial biopsy

Dilatation and curettage

The classic method of obtaining endometrium is by dilatation and curettage (D&C). This technique was first reported by Recamier in 1843 (cited in Ricci, 1949); he described the use of a small scoop attached to a long handle for removing intrauterine fungal growth and called this method curettage. This instrument was controversial until antiseptics were available; Recamier reported three deaths from its use as a result of perforation and subsequent peritonitis. Now D&C is one of the most common procedures performed and the rate in England was 71.1 per 10 000 in 1989–90 (Coulter et al, 1993). D&C is being increasingly replaced by outpatient procedures which avoid general anaesthesia and are also less costly. D&C is not without risk; perforation, haemorrhage and even mortality (Grimes, 1982). A D&C does not sample the whole of the endometrium. A study where curettage was performed pre-hysterectomy found that in 60% less than half of the cavity was curetted and in 16% less than a quarter (Stock and Kanbour, 1975). Since D&C is essentially a blind procedure it can miss lesions; in one study 6% of cases (polyps, hyperplasia and carcinoma) (Stovall et al, 1989).

Aspiration curettage

Vacuum or aspiration curettage was introduced in 1970. The first instru-ment was a 3 mm diameter stainless steel cannula with a curved tip and a wide slit on the concave surface attached to a plastic aspiration chamber and a vacuum (Jensen, 1974). Since then various types have been used with a plastic cannula (Rockett) which has either a 3 or 4 mm cannula. Suction can be generated either mechanically or electrically. More recently, internal piston suction devices have been devised (Pipelle, Wallach). They consist of a 3 mm plastic tube with an internal piston; its withdrawal after insertion into the uterine cavity generates suction pulling tissue into the cannula as it is rotated. The advantage of aspiration curettage is that it avoids general anaesthesia and has fewer complications than D&C (Grimes, 1982).

There have been many comparative studies of the different methods which support the use of outpatient aspiration curettage. Comparison of Vabra and D&C shows equal accuracy (Lutz et al, 1977; Grimes, 1982; Stovall et al, 1989). In the study by Stovall et al (1989) involving 619 women, there were no instances in which Vabra aspiration failed to discover carcinoma or a potentially pre-cancerous lesion; in two cases endometrial carcinoma was missed and in both D&C was the method of sampling.

Comparison of Pipelle and D&C in 187 women, showed both procedures had similar results in 164 women including detection of carcinoma; in the cases where there was discrepancy, no atypical hyperplasia or carcinoma were missed (Fothergill et al, 1992)

However, a comparison of Pipelle and Vabra, as measured by endometrial denudation in hysterectomy specimens, showed that the Pipelle sampled significantly less of the endometrial surface than the Vabra (Rodriguez et al, 1993). Here the percentage endometrial surface area sampled was 4.2% for the Pipelle and 41.6% for the Vabra. The number of endometrial surfaces sampled (one anterior and one posterior) were Pipelle 1 and Vabra 2. The mean number of endometrial quadrants sampled (four anterior plus four posterior) were Pipelle 2.4 and Vabra 7.4.

In contrast, a comparison of Pipelle and Novak curettage showed there was significantly less pain during the former than the latter procedure. In the patients who subsequently underwent hysterectomy, there was agreement in 96% between the pathological results of hysterectomy and those of endometrial samples (Stovall et al, 1991)

Endometrial cytology

Many studies have examined the possibility of evaluating the endometrium with cytology. A major limitation of this approach has been that a definitive diagnosis of cancer or hyperplasia cannot always be based on cytological findings (Chambers and Chambers, 1992). However, the finding of any endometrial cells on Papanicolaou smears from post-menopausal women dictates further evaluation as it is often related to endometrial disease.

Hysteroscopy

The hysteroscope provides direct visualisation of the endometrial cavity and was introduced over a century ago. Flexible, as well as rigid, hysteroscopes are now available. Some women require paracervical blocks for anaesthesia. It can be undertaken as an outpatient procedure. In a recent evaluation of 110 women with persistent post-menopausal bleeding, 40% had polyps, 50% had submucous fibroids and 2% had an adenocarcinoma (Townsend et al, 1993). Even hysteroscopy is not 100% accurate and in this series one adenocarcinoma was missed on initial evaluation.

Although the hysteroscopic evaluation of an endometrium is better able to identify endometrial polyps and submucous fibroids than endometrial biopsy, the necessity of hysteroscopy in all women with abnormal uterine bleeding has not yet been confirmed. Its place is best reserved for women with persistent bleeding where endometrial biopsy is negative or the endometrium abnormally thickened on ultrasound

Previous endometrial resection or ablation

We are now seeing an increasing number of women who have had a previous endometrial resection or ablation. Here the endometrial cavity may be partially obliterated, and assessment of the endometrium extremely problematic.

Transvaginal ultrasound

This technique is increasingly being used to evaluate the endometrium. A thickened endometrium or a cavity filled with fluid is suggestive of malignancy or other pathology (hyperplasia, polyps). Pre-menopausally, total anteroposterior thickness (both endometrial layers) varies from 4 to 8 mm in the proliferative phase and peaks at 8 to 16 mm during the secretory phase. In post-menopausal women, an endometrial thickness of less than 4 or 5 mm is suggestive of endometrial atrophy (Goldstein et al, 1990; Nasri et al, 1991; Varner et al, 1991). Endometrial thickness on cyclical HRT varies from 4 to 8 mm (Varner et al, 1991). Detection of endometrial polyps can be enhanced by instillation of contrast medium into the uterine cavity. It is debated whether vaginal ultrasound can replace endometrial biopsy. In one series, for example, the risk of finding pathological endometrium at curettage when the endometrium was less than 4 mm thick was 5.5% (Karlsson et al, 1995). However, it must be remembered that ultrasound does not give a histological diagnosis and cannot replace biopsy, but it is a useful adjunct when insufficient tissue is obtained (FDA HRT Working Group 1995).

SUMMARY

The endometrial effects of HRT are of prime importance in compliance with long-term use, and safety with therapy. Different regimens have to be advocated according to menopausal status, to produce acceptable bleeding patterns.

REFERENCES

Andersson K, Mattson LA, Rybo G & Stadberg E (1992) Intrauterine release of levonorgestrel—a new way of adding progestogen in hormone replacement therapy. *Obstetrics and Gynecology* **79:** 963–967.

Archer DF, McItyr-Seltman K, Wilborn WW et al (1991) Endometrial morphology in asymptomatic premenopausal women. *American Journal of Obstetrics and Gynecology* **65:** 317–322.

Archer DF, Pickar JH, Bottiglioni F for the Menopause Study Group (1994) Bleeding patterns in post menopausal women taking continuous combined or sequential regimens of conjugated oestrogens with medroxyprogesterone acetate. *Obstetrics and Gynecology* **83:** 686–692.

Barentsen R, Groenvaeld F, Bareman FP et al (1993) Women's opinion on withdrawal bleeding with hormone replacement therapy. *European Journal of Obstetrics and Gynecology and Reproductive Biology* **51:** 203–207.

Brinton L & Hoover R (1993) Estrogen replacement therapy and endometrial cancer: unresolved issues. *Obstetrics and Gynecology* **81:** 265–271.

Byrjalsen I, Thormann L, Riis BJ & Christiansen C (1992) Secretory endometrial protein PP14 in serum from postmenopausal women receiving continuous combined oestradiol-cyproterone acetate: correlation with serum hormone concentrations and bleeding patterns. *Maturitas* **15:** 39–46.

Casper RF & Chapdelaine A (1993) Estrogen and interrupted progestin: a new concept for menopausal hormone replacement therapy. *American Journal of Obstetrics and Gynecology* **168**: 1188–1194.

Chambers JT & Chambers SK (1992) Endometrial sampling: When? Where? Why? With What? *Clinical Obstetrics and Gynecology* **35**: 28–39.

Christiansen C & Riis BJ (1990) Five years with continuous combined oestrogen/progestogen therapy. Effects on calcium metabolism, lipoproteins and bleeding pattern. *British Journal of Obstetrics and Gynaecology* **97**: 1087–1092.

Cole SK, Billewicz WZ & Thomson AM (1971) Sources of variation in menstrual blood loss. *Journal of Obstetrics and Gynaecology of the British Commonwealth* **78**: 933–940.

Coope J & Marsh J (1992) Can we improve compliance with long-term HRT? *Maturitas* **15**: 151–158.

Coulter A, Klassen A, Mackenzie IZ & McPherson K (1993) Diagnostic dilatation and curettage: is it used appropriately? *British Medical Journal* **306**: 236–239.

Darj E, Axelsson O, Nilsson G et al (1995) Ki-67 immunostaining of endometrial biopsies with special reference to hormone replacment therapy. *Gynecology and Obstetric Investigation* **39**: 120–124.

David A, Czernobilsky B & Weisglass L (1993) Long-cyclic hormonal cycle therapy in post-menopausal women. In Berg G & Hammar M (eds) *The Modern Management of the Menopause.* pp 463–470. New York: Parthenon.

Ettinger B, Selby J, Citron J et al (1994) Cyclic hormone replacement therapy using quarterly progestin. *Obstetrics and Gynecology* **83**: 693–700.

FDA HRT Working Group (1995) Guidance for clinical evaluation of combination estrogen/progestin containing drug products used for hormone replacement therapy of postmenopausal women. *Menopause* **2**: 131–136.

Fothergill DJ, Brown VA & Hill AS (1992) Histological sampling of the endometrium—a comparison between formal curettage and Pipelle sampler. *British Journal of Obstetrics and Gynaecology* **99**: 779–780.

Fox H & Buckly CH (1982) The endometrial hyperplasia and their relationship to endometrial neo-plasia. *Histopathology* **4**: 493–510.

Fraser IS, McCarron G & Markham R (1984) A preliminary study of factors influencing perception of menstrual blood loss volume. *American Journal of Obstetrics and Gynecology* **149**: 788–793.

Gambrell RD (1978) The prevention of endometrial cancer in postmenopausal women with progestogens. *Maturitas* **1**: 99–106.

Gambrell R, Massey F, Castenada T et al (1980) Use of the progestogen challenge test to reduce the risk of endometrial cancer. *Obstetrics and Gynecology* **55**: 732–738.

Goldstein SR, Nachtigall M, Snyder JR & Nachtigall L (1990) Endometrial assessment by vaginal ultrasonography before endometrial sampling in patients with postmenopausal bleeding. *American Journal of Obstetrics and Gynecology* **163**: 119–123.

Grady D, Gebretsadik T, Kerlikowske K et al (1995) Hormone replacment therapy and endometrial cancer risk: a meta-analysis. *Obstetrics and Gynecology* **85**: 304–313.

Grimes DA (1982) Diagnostic dilatation and curettage; a reappraisal. *American Journal of Obstetrics and Gynecology* **142**: 1–15.

Grimwood J, Bicknell R & Rees MCP (1995) The isolation, characterization and culture of human decidual endothelium. *Human Reproduction* **10**: 2142–2148.

Hallberg L, Hogdahl AM, Nilsson I & Rybo G (1966) Menstrual blood loss—a population study. *Acta Obstetrica et Gynecologica Scandinavica* **45**: 320–351.

Hallberg L & Nilsson I (1964) Determination of menstrual blood loss. *Scandinavian Journal of Clinical and Laboratory Investigation* **16**: 244–248.

Hammond C, Jelovsek F, Lee K & Creasman W (1979) Effects of long term estrogen replacment therapy. II Neoplasia. *American Journal of Obstetrics and Gynecology* **133**: 537–547.

Hawthorn RJS, Spowart K, Walsh D & McKay Hart D (1991) The endometrial status of women on long term continuous combined hormone replacment therapy. *British Journal of Obstetrics and Gynaecology* **98**: 939–942.

Hirvonen E, Salmi T, Puolakka J et al (1995) Can progestin be limited to every third month only in postmenopausal women taking oestrogen? *Maturitas* **21**: 39–44.

Hope S & Rees M (1995) Why do British women start and stop HRT? *Journal of the British Menopause Society* **1**: 26–27.

Jensen JG (1970) Vacuum curettage. *Danish Medical Bulletin* **17:** 199–206.

Kaiserman-Abramof IR & Padykula HA (1989) Angiogenesis in the postovulatory primate endometrium: the coiled arteriolar system. *Anatomical Record* **224:** 479–489.

Karlsson B, Granberg S, Wikland M et al (1995) Transvaginal ultrasonography of the endometrium in women with postmenopasual bleeding—a Nordic study. *American Journal of Obstetrics and Gynecology* **172:** 1488–1494.

Kemp JF, Fryer JA & Baber RJ (1989) An alternative regimen of hormone replacement therapy to improve patient compliance. *Australian and New Zealand Journal of Obstetrics and Gynaecology* **29:** 66–69.

Koss LG, Schreiber K, Oberland SG et al (1984) Detection of endometrial carcinoma and hyperplasia in asymptomatic women. *Obstetrics and Gynecology* **64:** 1–11.

Kurman RJ, Kaminski PF & Norris HJ (1985) The behaviour of endometrial hyperplasia. A long term study of untreated hyperplasia in 170 patients. *Cancer* **56:** 403–412.

Lafferty FW & Fiske ME (1994) Postmenopausal estrogen replacment: a long term cohort study. *American Medical Journal* **97:** 66–77.

Leather AT, Savvas M & Studd JWW (1991) Endometrial histology and bleeding patterns after 8 years of continuous combined estrogen and progestogen therapy in postmenopasual women. *Obstetrics and Gynecology* **78:** 1008–1010.

Lutz MH, Underwood PB, Kreutner A & Mitchell KS (1977) Vacuum aspiration: an efficient out-patient screening technic for endometrial disease. *Southern Medical Journal* **70:** 393–399.

Markee JE (1940) Menstruation in intraocular endometrial transplants in the rhesus monkey. *Contributions to Embryology Carnegie Institution* **28:** 219–359.

Mishell DR, Shoupe D, Moyer DL et al (1991) Postmenopausal hormone replacment therapy with a combination estrogen-progestin regimen for 5 days per week. *Journal of Reproductive Medicine* **36:** 351–355.

Nasri MN, Shepherd JH, Setchell ME et al (1991) The role of vaginal scan in measurement of endometrial thickness in postmenopausal women. *British Journal of Obstetrics and Gynecology* **98:** 470–475.

Padwick M, Pryse-Davies J & Whitehead M (1986) A simple method for determining the optimal dosage of progestin in postmenopausal women receiving oestrogens *New England Journal of Medicine* **315:** 930–935.

Paterson MEL, Wade-Evans T, Sturdee DW et al (1980) Endometrial disease after treatment with oestrogens and progestogens in the climacteric. *British Medical Journal* **280:** 822–824.

Perrot-Applanat M, Groyer Picard M, Garcia E et al (1988) Immunocytochemical demonstration of oestrogen and progesterone receptors in muscle cells of uterine arteries in rabbits and humans. *Endocrinology* **123:** 1511–1519.

Persson I, Adami HO, Bergkvist L et al (1989) Risk of endometrial cancer after treatment with oestrogens alone or in conjunction with progestogens: results of a prospective study. *British Medical Journal* **298:** 147–151.

Rees MCP (1989) Heavy painful periods *Baillière's Clinical Obstetrics and Gynaecology* **3(2):** 341–356.

Rees MCP (1994) On menstrual bleeding with hormone replacement therapy. *Lancet* **343:** 250.

Rees MCP & Barlow DH (1991) Quantitation of hormone replacement induced withdrawal bleeds. *British Journal of Obstetrics and Gynaecology* **98:** 106–107.

Rees MCP & Sheppard B (1993) Endothelium ultrastructure of endometrium exposed to cyclical oestrogen progestogen replacement therapy. 7th International Congress on the Menopause. Abstract Book. p18.

Ricci JV (1949) *Gynaecologic Survey and Instruments of the Nineteenth Century Prior to the Antiseptic Age. The Development of Gynaecological Surgery and Instruments.* pp 326–328. Philadelphia, PA: Blakiston.

Rodriguez GC, Yaqub N & King ME (1993) A comparison of the Pipelle device and the Vabra aspirator as measured by endometrial denudation in hysterectomy specimens: the Pipelle samples significantly less of the endometrial surface than the Vabra aspirator. *American Journal of Obstetrics and Gynecology* **168:** 55–59.

Rusnati M, Casarotti G, Pecorelli S et al (1993) Estro-progestogenic replacement therapy modulates the levels of basic fibroblast growth factor (bFGF) in postmenopausal endometrium. *Gynaecological Oncology* **48:** 88–93.

Smith D, Prentice R, Thompson D & Hermann W (1975) Association of exogenous estrogen and endometrial carcinoma. *New England Journal of Medicine* **293:** 1164–1167.

Sporrong T, Rybo G, Mattson LA et al (1992) An objective and subjective assessment of uterine blood loss in postmenopausal women on hormone replacement therapy. *British Journal of Obstetrics and Gynaecology* **99:** 399–401.

Staland B (1981) Continuous treatment with natural oestrogens and progestogens. A method to avoid endometrial stimulation. *Maturitas* **3:** 145–156.

Stock RJ & Kanbour L (1975) A prehysterectomy curettage. *Obstetrics and Gyncecology* **45:** 537–560.

Stovall TG, Solomon SK & Ling FW (1989) Endometrial sampling prior to hysterectomy. *Obstetrics and Gynecology* **73:** 405–409.

Stovall TG, Ling FW & Morgan PL (1991) A prospective randomised comparison of the Pipelle endometrial sampling device with the Novak curette. *American Journal of Obstetrics and Gynecology* **165:** 1287–1289.

Sturdee DW, Barlow DH, Wells M et al (1994) Is the timing of withdrawal bleeding a guide to endometrial safety during sequential oestrogen-progestogen replacement therapy? *Lancet* **343:** 979–982.

Suhonen SP, Allonen HO & Lahteenmaki P (1995) Sustained-release estradiol implants and a levonorgestrel-releasing intrauterine device in hormone replacement therapy. *American Journal of Obstetrics and Gynecology* **172:** 562–567.

Townsend DE, Fields G, McCausland A & Kauffman K (1993) Diagnostic and operative hysteroscopy in the management of persistent postmenopausal bleeding. *Obstetrics and Gynecology* **82:** 419–421.

Udoff L, Langenberg P & Adashi EY (1995) Combined continuous therapy: a critical review. *Obstetrics and Gynecology* **86:** 306–316.

Varner RE, Sparks JM, Cameron CD et al (1991) Transvaginal sonography of the endometrium in postmenopausal women. *Obstetrics and Gynecology* **78:** 195–199.

Voigt L, Weiss N, Chu J et al (1991) Progestogen supplementation of exogenous oestrogens and risk of endometrial cancer. *Lancet* **338:** 274–277.

Williams DB, Voigt B, Fu YS, et al (1994) Assessment of less than monthly progestin therapy in postmenopausal women given estrogen replacement. *Obstetrics and Gynecology* **84:** 787–793.

Woodruff JD & Pickar JH for the Menopause Study Group (1994) Incidence of endometrial hyperplasis in postmenopausal women taking conjugated estrogens (Premarin) with medroxyprogesterone acetate or conjugated estrogens alone. *American Journal of Obstetrics and Gynecology* **170:** 1213–1232.

Zhang L, Rees MCP & Bicknell R (1995) The isolation and long-term culture of normal human endometrial epithelium and stroma. Expression of mRNAs for angiogenic polypeptides basally and on oestrogen and progesterone challenges. *Journal of Cell Science* **108:** 323–331.

6

The breast and the menopause

BARRY G. WREN

The breast is not only the source of nutrition for infants, of sexual arousal and gratification for both women and men, and an endocrine organ, but it is also a source of pain and discomfort for some women and the commonest site for cancer in females. As a consequence, any action or activity which involves the breast is of great concern not only to females but to their partners and to their family, friends and ultimately the whole community.

DEVELOPMENT, ANATOMY, PHYSIOLOGY AND BIOLOGY

The breast is composed of numerous cells with differing functions which may vary from secretory activity, duct formation and myoepithelial contraction to fat cells, nerve fibres, vascular supply and production of fibrous tissue and collagen. The breast is capable of functioning as a source of nutritious food and as an endocrine gland, controlling cellular activity within the breast independently of outside influence, yet capable of responding to messages produced elsewhere in the body.

Each breast is composed of millions of alveoli which have the capacity to secrete milk. Each alveolus is lined by a single layer of cells which, under the influence of specific hormones, is capable of producing milk which is secreted into the lumen of the alveolus. Contraction of myoepithelial cells then squeezes the milk into the collecting ducts which eventually pass to the nipple where 15 to 20 lacteals empty to the surface. The complex of alveolar cells, collecting ducts and myoepithelial cells is embedded in specialized fat cells through which pass the arteries, capillaries, veins, nerves and lymphatics. The fat cells in the breast have specialized functions including the ability to produce oestrogen locally (Blankenstein et al, 1992) as well as protecting delicate tissue within the breast. In young women, subject to the influence of a number of hormones including oestrogen and progestogen, the ducts and alveoli are relatively active and occupy a large portion of the total volume of the breast. Following the menopause, and withdrawal of sex hormones, the glands and ducts undergo atrophic changes so that the major proportion of breast cells are fat cells. For that reason, post-menopausal breast tissue appears relatively translucent to X-rays, except in those women where hormonal therapy has been used to maintain cellular, ductal and alveolar activity.

Baillière's Clinical Obstetrics and Gynaecology—
Vol. 10, No. 3, September 1996
ISBN 0–7020–2177–6
0950–3552/96/030433 + 15 $12.00/00

It is thought that breast tissue initially grows under the influence of oestrogen which stimulates the ducts to grow, extend and enlarge. However, the alveoli appear to require both oestrogen and progesterone to reach their full maturation. For this reason the breast is only fully developed and capable of mature function after a woman has begun to ovulate regularly. Secretion of milk, however, requires prolactin as well as the presence of insulin, thyroxine and cortisone to prime the mature alveolar cells. Release of oxytocin from the pituitary is required to complete the hormonal response of the breast to begin lactation.

The glands and ducts within the breast are not uniform in size, structure or response. Some glands and ducts may become grossly distended, while others are small and narrow in diameter. Although the gland shape is typically presented as being grape-like in structure, the glands are usually flattened, elongated and distorted. Some areas of the breast have numerous glands and ducts while other sites may have a preponderance of fat. Each breast cell has a finite span of activity before it undergoes apoptosis or further mitotic activity. This mitotic/apoptotic rate dictates a number of the anatomical changes within the breast as well as influencing the symptoms experienced or the potential to develop cancer.

It has long been known that oestrogen increases the rate of mitosis within both ductal and alveolar tissue. Meyer (1977), Masters et al (1977) and Going et al (1988) have examined breast cells in various phases of the menstrual cycle and have shown that during the follicular phase, there is a modest increase in mitosis within ductal cells but no great change within alveolar cells. The influence of progestogen on breast cells is much more controversial. Meyer (1977), Anderson et al (1982), Russo et al (1987) and Going et al (1988) have all demonstrated an increase in mitosis during the luteal (progesterone) phase of the menstrual cycle. Based on this information, it has been suggested that progestogens increase the risk of breast cancer (Key and Pike, 1988; Spicer and Pike, 1992; Pike et al, 1993). This hypothesis is supported by epidemiological studies (Ewertz, 1988; Bergkvist et al, 1989; Colditz et al, 1995). However, Musgrove et al (1991), Sutherland et al (1988), Clarke and Sutherland (1990) and Gompel et al (1986), hold differing views regarding the action of progestogens on breast cell activity. Musgrove et al (1991) in her elegant in vitro studies, has shown a biphasic activity of progestogens on breast cancer cells. Initially, progestogen increases the rate of mitosis in breast cells; this appears to occur following an increase in protein cyclins stimulating a surge in those breast cells passing from the late G1 phase of cell cycle activity into the S phase (Figures 1 and 2). However, within hours of the increase in cells entering mitosis, cell cycle activity is arrested in early G1 phase by the continued presence of progestogens (Figure 2). If this action is reproduced in vivo then the continual presence of progestogens should have an inhibitory effect on the rate of mitosis in breast cells and thus reduce the risk of spontaneous oncogenic mutations. Epidemiological studies where progestogen has been administered continuously in a medium–high dose would suggest that this is indeed so (Ewertz, 1988; Plu-Bureau et al, 1994; Eden et al, 1995; Wren and Eden, 1996).

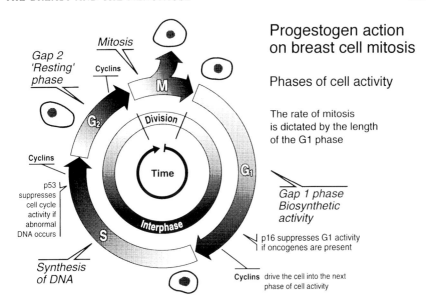

Figure 1. Diagrammatic representation of the four phases of cell activity. Progestogens initially induce a surge of cyclin activity in the late G1 phase but, within hours, cyclin production is reduced and cells are arrested in early G1 phase. G1 (Gap 1), protein biosynthetic phase; S, synthesis of DNA; G2 (Gap 2), resting phase; M, mitotic phase. Reproduced from Alberts et al (eds) (1989 *The Molecular Biology of the Cell*. p 728. New York: Garland Publishing) with permission.

While it would be tempting to suggest that all women receiving oestrogen therapy should be given progestogen in a continuous regimen, it is important to understand other biological actions of progestogen on breast cells.

Progestogens not only induce an initial surge in mitosis within hours of administration but also lead to changes in the alveolar cell cytoplasm. Cells begin to develop those changes which are associated with secretion of milk. There is an accumulation of fluid, electrolytes and proteins resulting in an increase in the size of the alveolar cell. Clinically, the initial effect of progesterone is to induce full, tender breasts for two to four weeks, but when no lactation occurs, the alveolar cells begin to undergo regression during which apoptosis exceeds mitosis. Over several weeks following continuous medium-dose progesterone activity, the breasts usually become smaller, less tense and less painful.

BREAST DISEASES

Breast cancer is the commonest malignancy among women, but the incidence varies considerably from country to country and race to race and is influenced by factors such as diet, parity and hormonal milieu. However, not every breast lump is cancerous and it is important to appreciate that

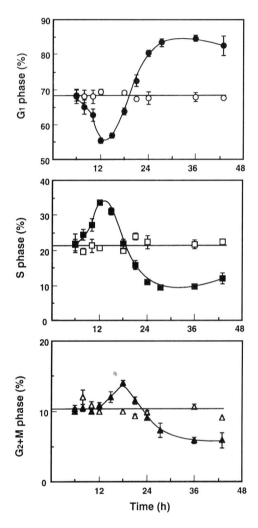

Figure 2. Effect of progestogen (ORG 2058) on breast cancer cell cycle phase distribution. An increase in the number of cells in the early part of S phase after 12 hours of treatment with progestogen is accompanied by a fall in cells in G1 phase. By 33 hours there is a marked decrease in S phase activity as well as a reduction in the number of cells in G2 and M phase. Under the influence of continuous progestogen cells remain in G1 phase. Reproduced from Musgrove et al (1991, *Molecular and Cellular Biology* **11**: 5032–5043) with permission.

most breast diseases are benign. The majority of lumps in breasts are discovered by the patient following self-exploration after an episode of pain or discomfort, and most women can be reassured that the mass is probably benign. However, every lump should be fully investigated. Initially palpation of a benign mass will usually disclose a firm or rubbery, mobile, tender area with a smooth outline not attached to the skin, nipple or underlying structures. While these findings suggest the area is benign, a mammographic examination should be performed and, if doubt still exists, an ultrasound review and fine-needle aspiration or core biopsy performed.

Benign breast tumours

Fibroadenosis, fibrocystic disease, hormonal mastopathy, hormonal mastitis or mammary dysplasia (Figure 3)

This group of synonyms is used to describe the commonest form of benign breast disease and accounts for over 90% of all breast lumps. The changes associated with fibroadenosis develop slowly over many months or years and become most evident in women between 35 and 55 years of age. It is caused by a proliferation of epithelial cells in the lobulo–alveolar region of the breast and is probably the result of cyclic oestrogen–progestogen acting on these cells. The overgrowth of epithelial cells results in an increase in papillary and polypoid tissue within ducts and alveoli, an increase in cystic dilatation of ducts and an increase in fibrosis and sclerosis in the surrounding stroma. The changes within the breast are not uniform and, within the same area of breast tissue, there may be dilated cysts and dense sclerosing fibrosis. It is almost certain that the disease is purely hormonal in origin resulting from oestrogen followed by intermittent progestogen activity. Ductal and lobulo–alveolar cells proliferate, resulting in overcrowding of the epithelium, causing cystic dilatation to some glands or ducts while others result in epithelial buckling and an increase in papillomas, polyps and nodules. The surrounding stroma responds to this proliferation by an

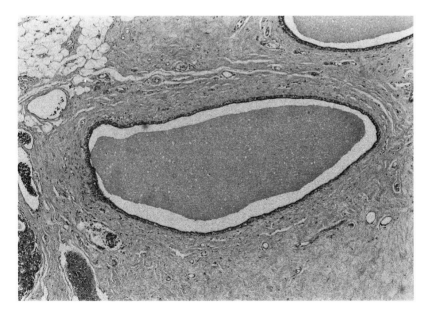

Figure 3. Fibroadenosis in breast tissue.

increase in fibrosis and sclerosis. While women are concerned about these discomforting hormonal changes, it is important to realize that there is no increased risk of breast cancer in these lumpy tender areas. Fibroadenosis does not increase the risk of cancer, however, because of the dense tissue, it becomes much more difficult to palpate a malignant mass. For that reason, detection of cancer may be delayed for some time resulting in an adverse outcome for the patient. Women with fibroadenosis should not have their hormonal therapy withdrawn but they should be warned to have regular palpation and mammography to ensure an early pick-up of abnormal changes.

Benign epithelial tumours

This group of diseases include intraduct papillomas, adenomas of the breast, adenomyoepitheliomas and adenomas of the nipple. These benign tumours are simple proliferative growths of the epithelial cells of the breast but may cause bleeding, pain or discharge. They should be excised when detected.

Mixed epithelial and connective tissue tumours

These tumours include fibroadenomas, cystosarcoma phyllodes, skin and soft tissue tumours (lipomas) and myoblastomas.

Other benign tumours

These include duct ectasia, inflammatory pseudotumours and hamartomas.

Aetiology and management of fibroadenosis

Oestrogen is responsible for the growth of duct epithelium while both oestrogen and progesterone are involved in the increased proliferation and secretory changes in lobulo–alveolar cells.

When there is so much proliferation and swelling within the breast that discomfort occurs women seek relief from a variety of means. Clearly, if cyclic oestrogen/progesterone are responsible for initiating the cellular changes which cause mastalgia, then hormones which reduce the pro-liferative/secretory changes will result in greatest relief and reversal of fibroadenosis and pain. However, without understanding the biological processes occurring in breast cells, many medical advisers have prescribed alternative therapies with only limited success.

It is important to realize that the breast is a dynamic organ with cells which respond to hormonal messengers to produce a variety of changes which markedly influence the size, structure, function and sensitivity of the breast. Not only will it respond to hormones but it is also capable of producing them in an autocrine manner which influence the dynamics of the breast. Blankenstein et al (1992) showed that breast fat cells are capable of aromatizing androgenic steroid precursors to produce levels of oestradiol up to 20 times greater than are present in circulating blood. This may explain why breasts produce localized changes which do not always reflect the levels of oestrogens acting on other sites in the body.

Oestrogen stimulates the production of both oestrogen and progesterone receptors in breast epithelial cells, whereas prolonged exposure to un-opposed progesterone depletes oestrogen and progesterone receptor pro-duction (Nardulli and Katzenellbogen, 1988). Continuous oestrogen acts to stimulate the ductal epithelium but the proliferation of these cells does not lead to severe pain. In older women whose breast epithelial tissue has become atrophic, there may be regeneration of cells in sufficient numbers to produce some fullness and discomfort with tingling in the nipples, but this mild mastalgia soon disappears. However, when progestogens are added to oestrogen in post-menopausal woman, there is an immediate response from lobulo–alveolar cells to produce a full, tense, tender breast. This mastalgia is so severe that some woman decide to cease hormonal therapy immediately and never re-initiate treatment.

MANAGEMENT OF POST-MENOPAUSAL MASTALGIA

Once it is appreciated how mastalgia occurs, steps can be taken to help alleviate the problem. Several options are available and all may be effective. In deciding on the course of action, the patients general wellbeing is paramount, and consideration should also be given to other symptoms and problems.

Ceasing hormonal therapy will, within a few days, result in a decrease in mastalgia and lead to a reduction in the size of the breast. Following remission of the breast pain, women should be counselled and advised as to the cause of the pain and how it can be controlled. Once the breast dis-comfort has subsided, then progestogen alone may be introduced. A medium–high dose progestogen will produce some minor discomfort for a week or so but as the level of both oestrogen and progesterone receptors is reduced, the breast cells rapidly undergo regression and apoptosis. When the breast feels soft again, then oestrogen can be administered, beginning with a low dose, gradually increasing till the appropriate level is achieved.

The disadvantage of this plan of management is that for some women progestogen results in bloating, weight gain and depression. If this occurs, then alternative regimens should be explored.

The administration of continuous medium–high dose unopposed progestogen will also achieve suppression of breast cell activity and this is another technique which can be employed to reduce mastalgia. Not only does progestogen reduce the level of receptors within ducts and alveoli but it appears to increase the rate of apoptosis. Within two to four weeks, breast tissue becomes softer and pain subsides. However, often the initial increase in cellular secretory change results in further discomfort and cessation of the therapy before it achieves its intended relief.

It is likely that this regimen of therapy exerts its action both locally and centrally. Medium dosage progestogen inhibits the hypothalamic–pituitary area and therefore reduces ovarian action as well as acting directly on breast cells to increase the death of cells, or to reduce the rate of mitosis. The use of intermittent or sequential progestogen therapy will however increase the mastalgia, by not only causing a surge of mitosis in the first few days of therapy, but by inducing a secretory change in the breast lobulo–alveolar cells. If unopposed progestogens are to be used, then the regimen must be continued for at least three months.

Danazol (Danocrine) is a synthetic androgen capable of suppressing the hypothalamic–pituitary axis. It probably has little or no direct action on the breast cells and its use to suppress mastalgia in the post-menopausal phase is not generally rewarding. Women who do use Danazol after the menopause often complain of unwelcome side effects including nausea, acne, oily skin and depressive mood changes. Its value in pre- and peri-menopausal women lies in its ability to suppress gonadotropins and thus eliminate the cyclic production of oestrogen and progestogen. The Cardiff group have used Danazol extensively and found it to be particularly useful in pre-menopausal women who complain of mastalgia; up to 70% of women gain relief (Gately and Mansell, 1990; Gately et al, 1992). However, there is no evidence the drug is of any benefit to post-menopausal women (Andrews, 1990).

Clomid (Clomiphene citrate) also suppresses the hypothalamic–pituitary axis and theoretically should inhibit the ovarian production of oestrogen and progestogen. However, it is not thought to have a direct action on breast tissue so is not recommended for the treatment of mastalgia in peri or post-menopausal women.

Bromocriptine mesylate (Bromocriptine) acts as a stimulant to dopamine receptors within the brain and thus inhibits the production of prolactin. Prolactin is necessary for the primed breast (oestrogen and progestogen influence) to induce lactation. By inhibiting prolactin in pre-menopausal women, there may be a considerable relief from mastalgia (Pye et al, 1985; Mansell and Dogliotti, 1990). However, in post-menopausal women, the use of Bromocriptine will not relieve the pain which has been caused by cyclic hormonal replacement therapy (HRT).

All plants including sunflower, canola, olives and the evening primrose contain essential fatty acids. These include linoleic acid and gammalinoleic acid which are thought to play some part in the production of prostaglandins. The use of Evening Primrose Oil has become popular to treat almost all symptoms arising in women but it has been used with a modicum of success in the management of mastalgia in both pre- and post-menopausal women (Pye et al, 1985). Without a firm biological basis to explain its action, some 40% of women claim that its use has improved their breast pain (Pye et al, 1985). As Evening Primrose Oil is harmless and has very few side effects, it is the preferred method of management for post-menopausal mastalgia when other forms of hormonal therapy have failed to work. The main drawback to Evening Primrose Oil is its cost, so it should clearly not be prescribed simply to substitute for a placebo.

Tamoxifen is an attenuated oestrogen which not only blocks the action of oestradiol but also stimulates the production of transforming growth factor β (TGF-β). When used in post-menopausal women with breast cancer, Tamoxifen has been associated with a relief of mastalgia. Fentiman et al (1988) used Tamoxifen in a clinical trial of 60 pre-menopausal women and found symptomatic relief in about 90%. It is likely that Tamoxifen acts locally on breast cells to not only block the action of oestrogen but also to increase the rate of apoptosis of cells.

Breast cancer

Hormones do not cause breast cancer but they may influence the rate of growth of cancer cells. Oestrogen increases the rate of mitosis while progestogens initially induce a surge in cell division before inhibiting cell mitosis (Sutherland et al, 1988; Clarke and Sutherland, 1990; Musgrove et al 1991) Tamoxifen inhibits breast cell mitosis by blocking the action of oestrogen as well as increasing breast cell production of TGF-β (Love and Koroltchouk 1993).

Breast cancer occurs as a result of a mutagenic transformation in DNA material during mitosis (Wren and Eden, 1996). While viral, chemical and radiation activity may be responsible for some mutagenic changes (inherited mutagens are thought to be responsible for up to 10% of cancers), spontaneous mutations are by far the most frequent antecedent to cancer. As women age, the fragmentation and mutation of DNA material becomes more evident. For this reason breast cancer is far more common over 70 years of age than under 40 years of age. The use of unopposed oestrogen or oestrogen with sequential or intermittent progestogen regimens increases the rate of mitosis, and therefore the increased risk of breast cancer rises with duration of use. There is now considerable epidemiological evidence to support this concept; a reported 20% increase in the incidence of breast cancer after five years of oestrogen use, a 40 to 50% increase after 10 years of oestrogen (or intermittent progestogen) therapy, and about a 70 to 80% increase after 20 years of unopposed oestrogen therapy (Ewertz, 1988; Bergkvist et al, 1989; Colditz et al, 1995). Those few long-term studies available where Tamoxifen, or continuous progestogens, have been used to oppose the mitotic influence of oestrogen, suggest that the use of these regimens reduces the risk of developing breast cancer (Ewertz, 1988; Early Breast Cancer Collaborative Group, 1992; Plu-Bureau et al, 1994; Eden et al, 1995).

It is estimated that from one to two million cells in a cluster are required to produce a sufficient mass to be detected on an X-ray or by palpation. Normally breast cancer cells double their number about once every three months so that for a single mutated cancer cell to develop a palpable mass requires from five to 10 years. The use of unopposed oestrogen may increase the mitotic rate so that a mass may be present in half that time. The use of progestogen in a continuous regimen however, may slow mitosis to the rate where the mass of cancer cells are not detected for 15 to 20 years. For some years, this inhibitory effect of progestogen has been utilized to slow the rate of progress of breast cancer following metastasis to distant sites (Madrigal et al, 1980; Pannuti et al, 1980; Robustelli de la Cuna et al,

1988). Now it is being advocated as a means of reducing the rate of development and growth of early breast cancer (Wren and Eden, 1996).

Clearly, every woman in the peri- and post-menopausal phases of her life should have a regular palpation of her breasts, should be encouraged to self-examine and should have regular mammography, ultrasound and, if indicated, a fine-needle biopsy of any suspicious mass. Lumpy breasts due to fibroadenosis are not pre-malignant and there is no increased risk of developing cancer. Women with lumpy breasts may require hormonal therapy if they suffer from symptoms of oestrogen deficiency but they should be encouraged to have an annual mammogram and regular palpation to determine whether any suspicious changes have developed.

Do hormones increase the risk of breast cancer?

The fear that hormones, administered to women in the post-menopausal phase, will induce an increase in breast cancer, is one of the major reasons given by women as to why they will not take hormonal therapy after the menopause. Because of this fear it is important that the information which is available regarding this risk is reviewed. While the incidence of breast cancer varies from country to country, race to race and diet to diet there appears to be several common features. The incidence of breast cancer is most common in females in a Western society who have had few children and who often delay the onset of child-bearing till later in life (Hulka, 1993; Mack, 1993). Japanese women who consume a diet high in phyto-oestrogens have a much lower risk of breast cancer than do Japanese women who live in a Westernized society where only small amounts of phyto-oestrogens are consumed.

A number of papers suggest that unopposed oestrogen, or oestrogen with sequential progestogens, increases the risk of breast cancer (Ewertz, 1988; Bergkvist et al, 1989; Colditz et al, 1995). Meta-analysis of a number of studies have, however, suggested that prolonged use of hormonal therapy is associated with a slight increase only, with the relative risk varying from 1.23 to 1.3 after seven to 14 years (Mack, 1993). More recently a paper by Colditz et al (1995) reviewed the data they had gathered from the Nurses Health Study. The Nurses Health Study was begun in 1976 when 121 700 female registered nurses in the USA, aged between 30 and 55 years, completed a mailed questionnaire. Every two years, a follow-up questionnaire was mailed to these women to ask them to update information on various risk factors including hormone usage. When any woman was identified as having breast cancer, a copy of the pathology report was obtained to confirm diagnosis. In 1976, 23 965 women were post-menopausal and this number had increased to 69 586 by 1990. Follow-up of individual women was terminated with the diagnosis of breast cancer, or on the death of the women or 1 June 1992. A proportional-hazards model was used to adjust for multiple risk factors in an attempt to correct for any biases. This type of analysis is regarded as a weak method compared to a prospective double-blind trial. However notwithstanding the inherent problems with the methodology, the results suggested there was an increased risk with the use of HRT. Overall, women who used HRT for more than five years had a relative risk of developing breast cancer of 1.54. Those women who used HRT for less than five years did not have any increased risk, while those women who had used hormones but had then ceased therapy some two to four years previously had a relative risk of only 0.80. This paper caused a considerable amount of media attention with headlines indicting oestrogen therapy as a cause for cancer, or statements by 'experts' that women who took hormonal therapy following the menopause had a 40 to 60% risk of suffering from breast cancer. Naturally, a number of women ceased taking their hormones. A paper was published within a month by Stanford et al (1995) which came to the conclusion that the use of oestrogen with progestogen for post-menopausal women did not appear to be associated with an increased risk of breast cancer, but this paper did not rate any media attention and the findings were ignored.

So, what is the risk, and how could the risk be affected by the use of hormones? During a woman's life-time she runs an 8% overall risk of developing breast cancer. During the 20 years following the menopause (50 to 70 years of age) about five women in every 100 will be found to suffer from breast cancer. An increased risk of 50% during that 20 years will result

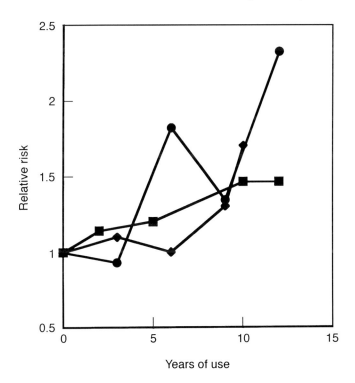

Figure 4. Graph illustrating the rising incidence of breast cancer with the prolonged use of unopposed oestrogen or oestrogen and sequential progestogen. —●—, Ewertz (1988); —◆—, Bergkvist et al (1989); —■—, Colditz et al (1995).

in seven or eight women having breast cancer; an increase of 2 to 3 only (not 50% as is often imagined by the press or women reading reports published in newspapers). It is likely that unopposed oestrogen, or oestrogen with sequential progestogen, increases the normal mitotic activity of ductal and lobulo-alveolar cells so that there would, in all likelihood, be an arithmetical increase in the rate of spontaneous chromosomal mutations. This should, over a period of some years, lead to an arithmetical increase of breast cancer; epidemiological studies confirm that this is so (Ewertz, 1988; Bergkvist et al, 1989; Colditz et al, 1995) (Figure 4).

It is also likely that hormones which slow the rate of cell division will result in a lower rate of chromosomal mutation and therefore a lowered risk of breast cancer. Hormones such as Tamoxifen and continuous progestogen usage have been shown to reduce the risk of developing breast cancer by 30 to 50% (Early Breast Cancer Collaborative Group 1992; Plu-Bureau et al, 1994; Eden et al, 1995) (Figure 5).

In conclusion, it can be stated that breast cancer is mostly a disease of post-menopausal women, that it increases with advancing age and the most common initiating cause is a chance spontaneous chromosomal mutation occurring during mitosis. Any factor which increases the rate of mitosis

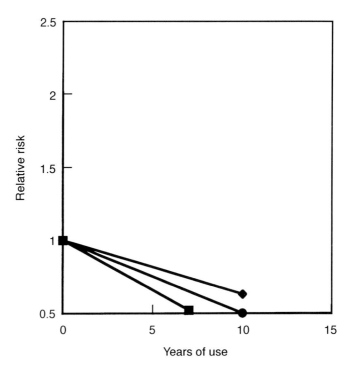

Figure 5. Graph illustrating the effect of continuous progestogen on the incidence of breast cancer in pre-menopausal women, and recurrences or new cases of cancer among women with a history of breast cancer. —◆—, Ewert (1988); —●—, Plu-Bureau et al (1994); —■—, Eden et al (1996).

(oestrogen) or is associated with easy fragmentation of chromosomal material (advancing age) will increase the risk of cancer. Factors which slow the rate of mitosis (withdrawal of oestrogens, use of Tamoxifen or continuous progestogen) will result in a lower rate of breast cancer.

Hormonal therapy following breast cancer

For many years the use of hormonal therapy following the discovery and treatment of breast cancer was thought to be contraindicated. However, a number of papers have now been published suggesting that, at least for stage I breast cancer, the use of oestrogen and progestogen following treatment of their cancer is not harmful (Stoll, 1989; Cobleigh et al, 1994; Eden et al, 1995). A large number of women are so severely affected by their oestrogen deficiency symptoms, that they are unable to function appropriately. The use of oestrogen for those patients taking HRT did not appear to have induced an adverse outcome, while in one study (Eden et al, 1995), the combined administration of oestrogen and medium-dose progestogen actually resulted in an improved long-term survival. Ninety women who suffered from symptoms of oestrogen deficiency following treatment for breast cancer were matched with 180 women with breast cancer who did not have hormonal therapy. Over a period of time averaging seven years of follow-up, the women receiving combined oestrogen and progestogen had half the rate of recurrence and no deaths when compared to matched controls. These results must be confirmed by further prospective studies.

REFERENCES

Alberts B, Bray D, Lewis J et al (eds) (1989) Cell growth and division. In *The Molecular Biology of the Cell*. 2nd edn, p 728. New York: Garland Publishing.

Anderson TJ, Ferguson DJ & Raab GM, (1982) Cell turnover in the 'resting' human breast: influence of parity, contraceptive pill, age and laterality. *British Journal of Cancer* **46**: 376–382.

Andrews WC (1990) Hormonal management of fibrocystic disease of the breast. *Journal of Reproductive Medicine* **35**: 87–90.

Bergkvist I, Adami H, Persson I et al (1989) The risk of breast cancer after estrogen and estrogen-progestogen replacement. *New England Journal of Medicine* **32**: 293–297.

Blankenstein MA, Szymczak J, Daroszewski J et al (1992) Estrogens in plasma and fatty tissue from breast cancer patients and women undergoing surgery for non-oncological reasons. *Gynaecological Endocrinology* **6**: 13–17.

Cobleigh MA, Berris RF, Bush T et al (1994) Estrogen replacement therapy in breast cancer survivors. Special Communications. *Journal of the American Medical Association* **272**: 540–545.

Colditz GA, Hankinson SE, Hunter DJ et al (1995) The use of estrogens and progestins and the risk of breast cancer in post menopausal women. *New England Journal of Medicine* **332**: 1589–1593.

Clarke CL & Sutherland RL (1990) Progestin regulation of cellular proliferation. *Endocrine Reviews* **11**: 266–301.

Early Breast Cancer Collaborative Group. (1992) Systemic treatment of early breast cancer by hormonal, cytoxic or immune therapy. Part 1. *Lancet* **339**: 1–15. Part 2 *Lancet* **339**: 71–85.

Eden JA, Bush T, Nand SL & Wren BG (1995) A case control study of combined continuous estrogen and estrogen-progestogen replacement therapy among women with a personal history of breast cancer. *Menopause* **2**: 67–72.

Ewertz M (1988) Influence of non-contraceptive exogenous and endogenous sex hormones on breast cancer risk in Denmark. *International Journal of Cancer* **42**: 832–838.

Fentiman IS, Caleffi M, Hamed H & Chaudry MA (1988) Dosage and direction of tamoxifen treatment for mastalgia: a controlled trial. *British Journal of Surgery* **75**: 845–846.

Gately CA & Mansell RE, (1990) Management of cyclical breast pain. *British Journal of Hospital Medicine* **43**: 330–332.

Gately CA, Miers M, Mansell RE & Hughes LE (1992) Drug treatments for mastalgia: 17 years experience in the Cardiff mastalgia clinic. *Journal of the Royal Society of Medicine* **85**: 12–15.

Going JJ, Anderson TJ, Battersby S & MacIntyre CCA (1988) Proliferative and secretory activity in human breast during natural and artificial menstrual cycles. *American Journal of Pathology* **139**: 193–204.

Gompell A, Malet C, Spritzer P et al (1986) Progestin effect on cell proliferation and 17β hydroxysteroid dehydrogenase activity in normal human breast cells in culture. *Journal of Clinical Endocrinology and Metabolism* **63**: 1174–1180.

Hulka BS, (1993) Hormonal risk factors for breast cancer. In Berg G & Hammer M (eds) *The Modern Management of the Menopause. Proceedings of the 7th International Congress on the Menopause.* pp 409–418. London: Parthenon.

Key TJA & Pike MC (1988). The role of oestrogens and progestogens in the epidemiology and prevention of breast cancer. *European Journal of Cancer and Clinical Oncology* **24**: 29–43.

Love RR & Koroltchouk V (1993) Tamoxifen therapy in breast cancer control world wide. *Bulletin of the World Health Organization* **71**: 795–804.

Mack TM (1993) Hormone replacement therapy and cancer. *Baillière's Clinical Endocrinology and Metabolism* **7**: 113–149.

Madrigal PL, Alouso A, Manga GP & Modrego SP (1980) High doses of medroxyprogesterone acetate (MPA) in the treatment of breast cancer. In Lacobelli S & Di Marco A (eds) *Role of Medroxyprogesterone in Endocrine Related Tumours.* pp 7–13. New York: Raven Press.

Mansell RE & Dogliotti L (1990) European multicentre trial on bromocryptine in clinical mastalgia. *Lancet* **335**: 190–193.

Masters JRW, Drife JO & Scarisbrick JJ (1977) Cycle variation of DNA in synthesis in human breast epithelium *Journal of the National Cancer Institute* **58**: 1263–1265.

Meyer JS (1977) Cell proliferation in normal human breast ducts, fibroadenosis, and other ductal hyperplasia measured by nuclear labelling with tritiated thymidine. Effects of menstrual phase, age, and oral contraceptive hormone. *Human Pathology* **8**: 67–81.

Musgrove E, Lee CSL & Sutherland RL (1991) Progestins both stimulate and inhibit breast expression of transforming growth factor α, epidermal growth factor receptor, c-fos and c-myc genes. *Molecular and Cellular Biology* **11**: 5032–5043.

Nardulli AM & Katzenellbogen BS (1988) Progesterone receptor regulation in T47D human breast cancer cells: analysis by density labelling of progesterone receptor synthesis and degradation on their modulation by progestin. *Endocrinology* **122**: 1532–1540.

Pannuti F, DiMarco AR & Marteni A (1980) Medroxyprogesterone acetate in treatment of metastatic breast cancer. Seven years experience. In Lacobelli S & Di Marco A (eds) *Role of Medroxyprogesterone in Endocrine Related Tumours.* pp 73–91. New York: Raven Press.

Pike MC, Spicer DV, Dahmoush L & Press MF (1993) Estrogens, progestins normal breast cell proliferation and breast cancer risk. *Epidemiological Reviews* **15**: 17–35.

Plu-Bureau G, Sitruk-Ware R, Thalabard JC & Mauvais-Jarvis P (1994) Progestogen use and the decreased risk of breast cancer in a cohort of pre-menstrual women with benign breast disease. *British Journal of Cancer* **70**: 270–277.

Pye JK, Mansell RE & Hughes LE (1985) Clinical experience of drug treatments for mastalgia. *Lancet* **ii**: 373–377.

Robustelli de la Cuna G, Pavesi L, Preti P & Baroni M (1988) High doses of medroxyprogesterone acetate in breast cancer, controlled studies. *Advances in Clinical Oncology* **1**: 45–46.

Russo J, Calaf G, Roi L & Russo IH (1987) Influence of age and gland topography on cell kinetics of normal human breast tissue. *Journal of the National Cancer Institute* **78**: 413–418.

Spicer DV & Pike MC (1992) The prevention of breast cancer through reduced ovarian steroid exposure. *Acta Oncologica* **31**: 167–174.

Stanford JL, Weiss NS, Voigt LF et al (1995) Combined estrogen and progestin hormone replacement therapy in relation to risk of breast cancer in middle aged women. *Journal of the American Medical Association* **274**: 137–142.

Stoll BA (1989) Hormonal replacement therapy in women treated for breast cancer. *European Journal of Clinical Oncology* **25**: 1909–1913.

Sutherland RL, Hall RE, Pang GYN et al (1988) Effect of medroxyprogesterone acetate on pro-
    liferation and cell cycle kinetics of human mammary carcinoma cells. *Cancer Research* **48:**
    5084–5091.
Wren BG & Eden JA (1996) Do progestogens reduce the risk of breast cancer? A review of the
    evidence. *Menopause* **3:** 4–12.

7

Metabolic effects of the menopause and oestrogen replacement

JOHN C. STEVENSON

Cardiovascular disease incidence increases with age in women as well as in men, but in women there is an additional increase due to the menopause (Gordon et al, 1978). Indeed, women have a 3.4-fold increase in risk of atherosclerosis after a natural menopause (Witteman et al, 1989). Cardiovascular disease is the leading cause of death in women, but these deaths occur at a later age than in men. This is perhaps why the importance of female coronary heart disease (CHD) in terms of morbidity and mortality is often overlooked. Although cardiovascular mortality is 2.7 times greater in males than in females below age 55, over all ages it is almost as high in females as in males in the UK. In the USA, mortality from CHD is now greater in women. Although death cannot be postponed indefinitely, prevention of premature mortality and particularly compression of morbidity (Freis et al, 1989) should be our primary aims in health care.

With regard to morbidity, the prevalence of angina is greater in women than in men over the age of 35 (LaCroix et al, 1989). This prevalence of angina includes cases of syndrome X—anginal chest pain, a positive ECG exercise test but no abnormality seen on coronary angiography (Kemp et al, 1973). Syndrome X occurs more frequently in women than in men.

MENOPAUSE AND RISK FACTORS FOR CHD

Whilst some metabolic risk factors for CHD in males have been defined, little is known of the relevance of these factors to the onset of CHD in females. Traditional CHD risk factors such as smoking, hypertension and hyperlipidaemia appear as important in older women as in younger men (Wilhelmsen et al, 1977), but less than half of the incidence of CHD is accounted for by these established risk factors in men (Kannel, 1982) and perhaps only a third in women. Thus the importance of other factors is becoming increasingly realised. Ovarian failure clearly leads to an increase in cardiovascular disease in women (Oliver and Boyd, 1959;

Baillière's Clinical Obstetrics and Gynaecology —
Vol. 10, No. 3, September 1996
ISBN 0–7020–2177–6
0950–3552/96/030449 + 19 $12.00/00

Sznajderman and Oliver, 1963; Gordon et al, 1978). Loss of ovarian function results in an increase in various CHD risk factors which appear to form a metabolic syndrome. These include adverse changes in lipids and lipoproteins, glucose and insulin metabolism, body fat distribution, coagulation and fibrinolysis, an increase in uric acid and a deterioration in vascular endothelial function. There appears to be a clustering of metabolic risk factors in patients with CHD, and it has been proposed that insulin resistance and hyperinsulinaemia are pivotal disturbances (Reaven, 1988). Hormone replacement therapy (HRT) might therefore be expected to reverse these changes, thereby reducing the increased cardiovascular disease risk.

GLUCOSE AND INSULIN METABOLISM

Diabetic women have a higher incidence of CHD than diabetic men (Abbott et al, 1987), demonstrating that women are more adversely affected by diabetes. Thus the effects of sex hormone deficiency and replacement on glucose and insulin metabolism may be of considerable importance. Furthermore, lesser degrees of glucose intolerance are predictive of subsequent CHD (Welborn and Wearne, 1979; Jarrett et al, 1982; Fuller et al, 1983; Donahue et al,1987). Protein glycosylation is a possible mechanism linking elevated glucose levels with CHD in diabetics, but the increased risk seen in those with lesser degrees of glucose tolerance are more likely to be mediated through insulin resistance and hyperinsulinaemia. Elevated insulin concentrations are frequently found in both men and women with CHD (Rönnemaa et al, 1991; Ley et al, 1994), and appear to be due to insulin resistance (Ley et al, 1994). We have also demonstrated increased insulin resistance in both men (Swan et al, 1994) and women (Godsland et al, 1995) with syndrome X.

Hyperinsulinaemia may increase CHD risk by directly promoting atherogenesis (Stout, 1990), and insulin propeptides may be of importance in this respect (Båvenholm et al, 1995). However, increased insulin concentrations may adversely affect several other CHD risk factors. There is an association between hyperinsulinaemia and hypertension (Ferrannini et al, 1987), and we have found a positive relationship between insulin resistance and blood pressure (Ley et al, 1994).

Insulin resistance and hyperinsulinaemia are also related to adverse changes in lipids and lipoproteins such as increased triglycerides and reduced high density lipoproteins (HDL) or HDL_2 concentrations (Ley et al, 1994). Furthermore, hyperinsulinaemia is associated with increased proportions of small dense low density lipoproteins (LDL) (Krauss, 1991). This association of adverse CHD risk factors is now termed the insulin resistance syndrome, and there are certain other components (Table 1). These include increased levels of the anti-fibrinolytic plasminogen activator inhibitor-1 (PAI-1) (Juhan-Vague et al, 1989), and increased proportions of android (central or upper body segment) fat (Stevenson et al, 1990).

Table 1. Established and postulated associations of the insulin resistance syndrome.

- Insulin resistance
- Hyperinsulinaemia
- Increased proportion of insulin propeptides
- Impaired glucose tolerance
- Increased triglycerides
- Decreased HDL and HDL_2 cholesterol
- Increased proportion of LDL cholesterol subtype B
- Increased proportion of android fat
- Increased NEFA flux
- Hyperuricaemia
- Increased plasminogen activator inhibitor-1
- Decreased arterial wall compliance
- Increased blood pressure
- Decreased arterial blood flow

HDL = high density lipoproteins, LDL = low density lipoproteins, NEFA = non-esterified fatty acids.

Effect of menopause on glucose and insulin metabolism

Few studies have investigated changes in glucose and insulin metabolism in relation to the menopause. One longitudinal study of women going through natural menopause showed increases in fasting glucose and insulin concentrations, but these were also seen in those women who remained pre-menopausal, suggesting an effect of ageing (Matthews et al, 1989). We have investigated glucose and insulin metabolism in a study of 86 healthy post-menopausal women who underwent an intravenous glucose tolerance test with measurement of glucose, insulin and C-peptide concentrations (Proudler et al, 1992). No relationship was seen between either chronological age or menopausal age and any glucose or C-peptide parameters, although body mass index was related to fasting glucose and post-glucose challenge glucose area. We found a positive and independent relationship between menopausal age and fasting insulin concentration and post-glucose challenge area, but no relation of these parameters with chronological age. This demonstrates that there is a progressive rise in insulin concentrations and responses to glucose challenge following the menopause. Further clarification of these findings resulted from another study of 158 pre- and post-menopausal women. In this study we performed mathematical modelling analyses of the plasma concentration profiles of glucose, insulin and C-peptide in response to an intravenous glucose challenge to obtain measures of insulin sensitivity, secretion and elimination (Walton et al, 1993). We found that post-menopausal women had a reduction in pancreatic insulin secretion which was counterbalanced by a reduction in insulin elimination (Figure 1). Insulin resistance increased progressively with age in the post-menopausal women (Figure 2).

It would thus appear that the menopause is associated with reduced pancreatic insulin secretion but with reduced insulin elimination, thereby

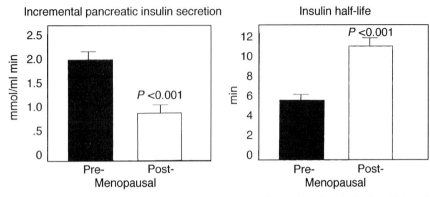

Figure 1. Effects of menopause on pancreatic insulin secretion and insulin elimination. (Adapted from Walton et al, 1993.)

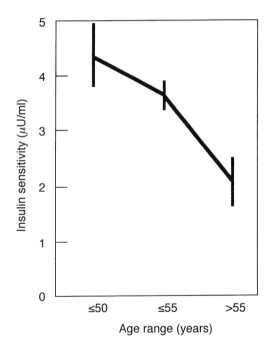

Figure 2. Effect of age on insulin sensitivity in post-menopausal women. (Adapted from Walton et al, 1993.)

resulting in little change in circulating insulin concentrations. The progressive rise in insulin concentrations thereafter appears to result from the progressive increase in insulin resistance seen after the menopause. Post-menopausal women thus become increasingly insulin resistant and hyperinsulinaemic.

HRT effects on glucose and insulin metabolism

Experimental studies both in vitro and in vivo have demonstrated increased pancreatic insulin secretion in response to oestrogen or progesterone administration. However, whilst oestrogen decreases insulin resistance, progesterone appears to increase it.

Clinical studies of the effects of oestradiol-17β in post-menopausal women suggest an improvement in insulin resistance (Notelovitz et al, 1987; Cagnacci et al, 1992). In contrast, alkylated oestrogens such as ethinyl oestradiol and conjugated equine oestrogens may raise insulin levels and impair glucose tolerance (Spellacy et al, 1972). Progestogen addition, which is necessary in HRT given to non-hysterectomized women, may produce certain adverse effects on glucose and insulin metabolism. We have performed a study in healthy post-menopausal women comparing two different HRT regimens against no treatment (Godsland et al, 1993). One regimen used oral conjugated equine oestrogens 0.625 mg daily with the cyclical addition of *dl*-norgestrel 0.15 mg daily whilst the other comprised transdermal oestradiol-17β 0.05 mg daily together with cyclical norethisterone acetate 0.25 mg daily. Transdermal treatment had no significant effect on glucose tolerance or insulin concentrations. In contrast, oral therapy caused a reduction in the initial plasma insulin response to intravenous glucose (Figure 3) which in turn resulted in a reduction in glucose elimination rate at the outset of the test and an overall elevation in glucose concentrations. These changes increased the stimulation of pancreatic

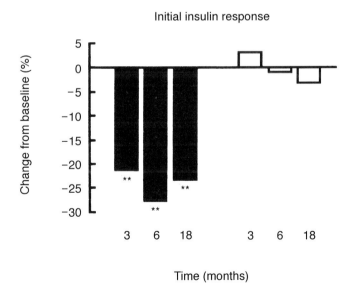

Figure 3. Initial plasma insulin response to a glucose challenge in post-menopausal women receiving either transdermal oestradiol-17β 0.05 mg daily with cyclical transdermal norethisterone acetate 0.25 mg daily (□), or oral conjugated equine oestrogens 0.625 mg daily with cyclical oral *dl*-norgestrel 0.15 mg daily (■) (**$P < 0.01$). (Adapted from Godsland et al, 1993.)

insulin secretion and hence the overall insulin response during the test (Figure 4). Both treatments were associated with increased hepatic insulin uptake, but an increase in first phase pancreatic insulin secretion compensated for this in the transdermal group. In the oral group, a significant increase in insulin resistance was seen during the combined oestrogen/progestogen phase of treatment compared with the oestrogen alone phase. The fact that transdermal oestradiol-17β was not associated with a reduction in insulin resistance, which might have been expected, could have been due to such an effect being negated by the norethisterone acetate, with a carry-over of this negative effect of norethisterone acetate into the oestrogen alone phase of treatment.

The use of a non-androgenic progestogen may avoid these adverse changes in glucose and insulin metabolism. We have studied the effects of oral administration of oestradiol-17β and cyclical dydrogesterone on glucose and insulin metabolism using oral glucose tolerance testing. Mean fasting glucose and C-peptide concentrations and post-glucose challenge incremental glucose and C-peptide areas remained unchanged during the study, whilst the fasting insulin concentration and post-glucose challenge response fell significantly (Crook et al, submitted). These findings are consistent with an improvement in insulin resistance and insulin elimination with this regimen.

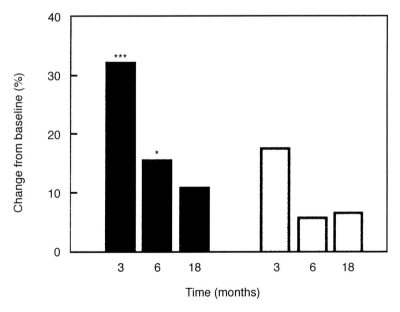

Figure 4. Phase 2 insulin response to a glucose challenge in post-menopausal women receiving either transdermal oestradiol-17β 0.05 mg daily with cyclical transdermal norethisterone acetate 0.25 mg daily (□), or oral conjugated equine oestrogens 0.625 mg daily with cyclical oral dl-norgestrel 0.15 mg daily (■) (*P < 0.05; ***P < 0.001). (Adapted from Godsland et al, 1993).

LIPIDS AND LIPOPROTEINS

It is well established that high circulating levels of cholesterol are associated with an increased incidence of CHD. LDL account for the major portion of total plasma cholesterol in most individuals and increased concentrations of LDL cholesterol lead to an increased risk of CHD. However, whilst the lowering of LDL cholesterol concentrations in men reduces the risk of CHD, it is not clear that the same effect can be achieved in women. The clearance of LDL and the intermediate density lipoproteins (IDL) from the circulation is effected by hepatic receptors. This process is slow and operates at near saturation of the receptors (Krauss, 1991). Thus if LDL concentrations are high, the LDL will have a relatively long half-life in the circulation. This makes them more susceptible to modification or damage, and damaged LDL are more likely to be retained intramurally in the arteries. Post-prandial lipoprotein remnants are also atherogenic and thus the efficiency of the clearance of such remnants is also important.

LDL comprises various subclasses differing in size, chemical composition and density (Shen et al, 1981). Lipoprotein (a) is an LDL which contains two distinct apoplipoproteins, apolipoprotein B and apolipoprotein (a). The latter is structurally a giant mutant of plasminogen (Utermann, 1989). It has been suggested that lipoprotein (a) is an independent lipoprotein risk marker for CHD, with high levels being associated with an increased risk of CHD. However, this is not an invariable finding and it may be that high lipoprotein (a) concentrations signify an increased CHD risk only when LDL levels are also raised. Lipoprotein (a) is atherogenic largely because of its propensity for retention in the arterial wall. It binds avidly to arterial proteoglycans (Dahlén et al, 1978), and also enhances arterial LDL retention (Yashiro et al, 1993). Lipoprotein (a) is also potentially thrombogenic because of its structural homology with plasminogen. It may thus compete with plasminogen for binding sites and inhibit fibrinolysis, and it also binds fibrin (Loscalzo et al, 1990).

LDL particle size varies and can be classified into subgroups accordingly. It has been shown that LDL particle size is clinically important. Patients with CHD, and particularly female patients, have an increased proportion of small dense LDL compared with healthy controls (Austin et al, 1988), a pattern described as subtype B. These smaller denser LDL particles are more atherogenic, perhaps because they are more readily cleared through scavenger mechanisms rather than by the $apoB_{100}$ receptors, and also because they may be more susceptible to oxidative damage (Tribble et al, 1992). Small dense LDL are found in individuals with raised triglycerides and low HDL (Austin et al, 1988) and are a feature of the metabolic syndrome (Reaven et al, 1993).

HDL may participate in reverse cholesterol transport whereby they remove cholesterol from tissues such as arterial walls and return it to the liver for excretion or resecretion. Thus HDL levels are inversely associated with CHD risk (Miller, 1987), with high levels considered to be protective. The HDL_2 subfraction is considered to be the subfraction which confers the major benefit, and HDL_2 can be catabolized by hepatic lipase. Conditions which increase hepatic lipase activity, such as increased adiposity or increased androgen activity, are associated with low HDL$_2$ levels. Triglyceride levels are inversely associated with HDL and HDL$_2$ levels (Stevenson et al, 1993). Increased hepatic triglyceride production leads to increased levels of triglyceride-rich very low density lipoproteins (VLDL). Reduced VLDL clearance results in increased plasma residence of VLDL remnants, decreased HDL$_2$ and increased IDL levels (Krauss, 1991), an atherogenic lipoprotein profile. Thus low levels of HDL and HDL$_2$ may reflect a reduction in reverse cholesterol transport or a reduction in VLDL remnant clearance, and it is not clear which is more important. The role of the HDL$_3$ cholesterol subfraction is less clear. Animal model studies have shown that increased levels of apolipoprotein AI are associated with a decrease in the development of vascular fatty streaks (Rubin et al, 1991) whereas increased levels of apolipoprotein AII are associated with an increase in their development (Mahrabian et al, 1993; Warden et al, 1993). In humans, an increase in apolipoprotein AII would be associated more with an increase in HDL$_3$ whereas an increase in apolipoprotein AI would be associated more with an increase in HDL$_2$ concentrations. It therefore remains possible that high levels of HDL$_3$, in contrast to HDL$_2$, are disadvantageous in terms of CHD risk.

Several processes have been implicated in the initiation of atheromatous lesions, including endothelial injury or increased permeability, and turbulent blood flow causing sheer stress-induced endothelial alteration. A unifying hypothesis for the development of atherosclerotic lesions has been postulated (Williams and Tabas, 1995) which suggests that the initial and most important event is subendothelial retention of atherogenic lipoproteins (Figure 5). Arterial proteoglycans, together with lipoprotein lipase and sphingomyelinase, are largely responsible for the intramural retention

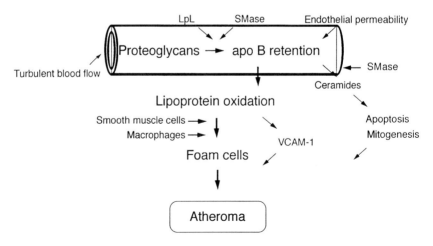

Figure 5. Retention of lipoprotein hypothesis as the initiating event in the formation of atheroma. SMase, sphingomyelinase; LpL, lipoprotein lipase. (Adapted from Williams and Tabas, 1995.)

of LDL and particularly lipoprotein (a), and these retained lipoproteins have increased sensitivity to oxidation. Oxidized lipoproteins are chemo-attractive to monocytes, smooth muscle cells and T-lymphocytes, and are avidly taken up to form foam cells which then progress to the development of the atheromatous plaque. Alterations in endothelial permeability, such as are seen in smoking and in dyslipidaemias, may contribute to this process, and sheer stress from turbulent blood flow may also induce lipoprotein retention by stimulating proteoglycans synthesis. The factors responsible for the focal retention of lipoproteins, and hence subsequent lesion development, are still not established.

Effects of menopause on lipids and lipoproteins

Whilst profound effects of exogenous sex steroids on lipids and lipoproteins have been demonstrated, there has been more controversy about the effects of endogenous female hormones. This is partly due to the fact that age and menopause are closely related, and many cross-sectional studies have not included sufficient numbers or a wide enough age range to permit the age adjustments necessary to determine any independent effects of the menopause. Furthermore, menopausal status has often not been adequately determined, and studies of pre- and post-menopausal women around the age of the menopause will inevitably be confounded by the inclusion of peri-menopausal women of similar hormonal status in both groups. The use of women with premature menopause who can be matched with pre-menopausal controls may be invalid as the former are not representative of the normal population. Equally, studies of women undergoing surgical menopause can be confounded by the catabolic effects of the surgery itself.

We have measured lipids and lipoproteins in a large cross-sectional study of 542 healthy non-obese Caucasian females aged between 18 and 70 years (Stevenson et al, 1993). Pre-menopausal status was defined by a regular menstrual cycle whilst post-menopausal status was defined by amenorrhoea and elevated gonadotrophins. In order to study the effects of the menopause independently of age, multiple linear regression analyses were performed separately for the pre- and post-menopausal women and these were used to standardize for confounding variables such as chronological age, and anthropometric and lifestyle parameters. We found that the standardized mean values for total cholesterol and triglycerides, LDL and HDL_3 cholesterol were significantly higher in post-menopausal women whilst those of HDL and particularly HDL_2 cholesterol were significantly lower (Figure 6). Our findings are in agreement with longitudinal studies (Matthews et al, 1989; Jensen et al, 1990). A further analysis of one of these studies (Kuller et al, 1990) demonstrated the striking effect of the menopause on HDL_2 cholesterol, in accordance with our findings. These various changes in lipids and lipoproteins should be regarded as potentially detrimental in terms of CHD risk.

Other adverse changes include a reported increase in lipoprotein (a) (Meilahn et al, 1991) and a shift in LDL particle size towards smaller denser LDL (Campos et al, 1988).

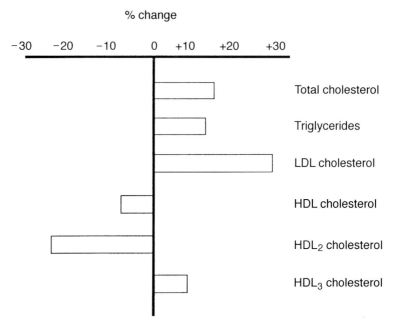

Figure 6. Effect of menopause on lipids and lipoproteins. LDL, low density lipoproteins; HDL, high density lipoproteins. (Adapted from Stevenson et al, 1993.)

Effects of HRT on lipids and lipoproteins

The effects of HRT on lipids and lipoproteins will depend on the particular type of oestrogen given, its dose and its route of administration. These effects may be modified if a progestogen is added as part of the HRT, again depending on the particular type of progestogen used, its dose and its route of administration. Progestogen effects may also depend on the regimen employed, so that the effects may be more pronounced if the total dose of the progestogen given is higher, such as by using it in a continuous rather than a cyclical fashion.

It is well established that oestrogen lowers total cholesterol, irrespective of the type of steroid or route of administration (Figure 7), and this effect is maintained in the long term whilst on treatment (Whitcroft et al, 1994). This lowering of cholesterol results primarily from a decrease in LDL cholesterol concentrations due to an up-regulation of $apoB_{100}$ receptors. The greatest magnitude of decrease in LDL with HRT appears to be seen in those with the highest baseline levels (Tikkanen et al, 1979). HRT may therefore be considered as a lipid-lowering agent in post-menopausal women with mild to moderate hypercholesterolaemia.

Oestrogen may reduce the levels of lipoprotein (a), although such an effect appears rather small and has not been extensively studied. Qualitative changes in LDL induced by HRT may also be of relevance. HRT appears to increase the proportion of small dense LDL particles (van

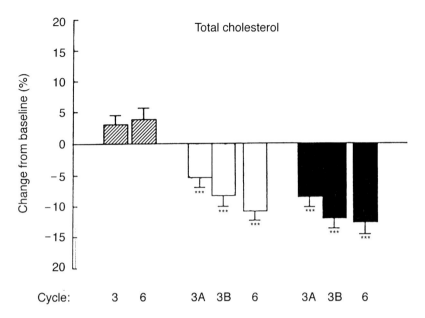

Figure 7. Changes in total cholesterol in post-menopausal women receiving either no treatment ▨, transdermal oestradiol-17β 0.05 mg daily with cyclical transdermal norethisterone acetate 0.25 mg daily (▢), or oral conjugated equine oestrogens 0.625 mg daily with cyclical oral *dl*-norgestrel 0.15 mg daily (■). 3A, oestrogen alone phase; 3B, combined phase; 6, combined phase. (***P <0.001). (Adapted from Crook et al, 1992a.)

der Mooren et al, 1994). This finding would appear to be somewhat paradoxical in view of the known lowering of CHD risk seen with HRT. However, other studies have suggested that HRT in fact decreases the proportion of larger LDL particles (Campos et al, 1993), and particularly IDL cholesterol (Westerveld et al, 1995), thus this change in LDL subtype pattern is not necessarily adverse. Oestrogen appears to protect against lipoprotein oxidation, thereby rendering the LDL less atherogenic (Sack et al, 1994), and also improves the post-prandial clearance of potentially atherogenic lipoprotein remnants (Westerveld et al, 1995).

Orally administered oestrogen increases HDL cholesterol, and particularly the HDL_2 subfraction which is thought to confer a protective effect against atherosclerosis development, by inhibiting hepatic lipase activity and by increasing the hepatic synthesis of apolipoprotein AI. Transdermal oestradiol appears to have a less marked effect on HDL cholesterol (Crook et al, 1992a) (Figure 8). However, although it may cause little increase in HDL_2, it does cause a reduction in HDL_3 which, as stated above, could itself be a theoretically beneficial effect for CHD risk.

The type and route of administration of oestrogen determines its effects on triglycerides. As triglycerides appear to be a particular risk factor for CHD in women (Bengtsson et al, 1993), this is of potential importance. Conjugated equine oestrogens cause an increase in triglycerides (Crook et

460 J. C. STEVENSON

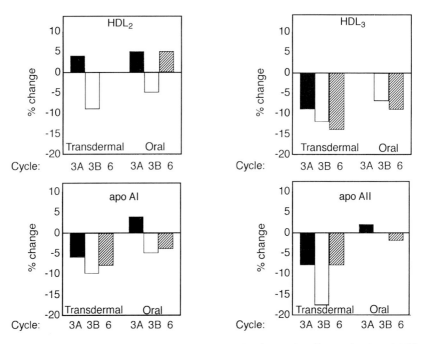

Figure 8. Changes in high density lipoprotein (HDL) subfractions and apolipoproteins AI and AII in post-menopausal women receiving either transdermal oestradiol-17β 0.05 mg daily with cyclical transdermal norethisterone acetate 0.25 mg daily, or oral conjugated equine oestrogens 0.625 mg daily with cyclical oral *dl*-norgestrel 0.15 mg daily. 3A, oestrogen alone phase; 3B, combined phase; 6, combined phases (**$P < 0.01$; ***$P < 0.001$). (Adapted from Crook et al, 1992a.)

al, 1992a), an effect which is pharmacological resulting from the hepatic first-pass effect of this steroid. Orally administered oestradiol has little or no effect on raising triglycerides, but transdermal oestradiol causes a reduction in triglycerides (Crook et al, 1992a) which is the physiological effect of oestrogen (Figure 9).

Progestogens have differing effects on lipids and lipoproteins, depending more on their androgenicity and perhaps dose duration rather than their route of administration. The addition of progestogens to oestrogen therapy has no obvious adverse effect in terms of lowering of LDL, since they increase LDL production but also increase their clearance (Wolfe and Huff, 1993). Androgenic progestogens, such as norgestrel, reverse the HDL-raising effect of oestrogen (Crook et al, 1992a) because they increase hepatic lipase activity. This effect is regarded as potentially disadvantageous, although it is most pronounced in patients with high HDL$_2$ levels and paradoxically may not occur in those with low HDL$_2$ levels (Stevenson, 1995). Thus, similar to the effects of HRT on LDL, patients with the greatest dispersions from normal in HDL$_2$ concentrations may show the most beneficial response in changes seen with HRT. Since it is not known whether the reduction in HDL reflects any impairment in remnant clearance, the clinical significance of lowering HDL remains to be determined. Androgenic compounds also lower lipoprotein (a) (Farrish et al, 1991; Crook et al, 1992b; Rymer et al, 1993; Marsh et al, 1994) (Figure 10), an effect which might be beneficial. In contrast, the less androgenic progestogens do not impede the oestrogen-induced increase in HDL cholesterol to any great extent but may not lower lipoprotein (a). The effect of progestogens on lipoprotein oxidation is currently unknown.

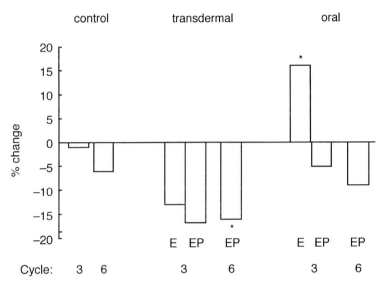

Figure 9. Changes in triglycerides in post-menopausal women receiving either no treatment, transdermal oestradiol-17β 0.05 mg daily with cyclical transdermal norethisterone acetate 0.25 mg daily, or oral conjugated equine oestrogens 0.625 mg daily with cyclical oral *dl*-norgestrel 0.15 mg daily. 3A, oestrogen alone phase; 3B, combined phase; 6, combined phase. (*$P < 0.05$). (Adapted from Crook et al, 1992a.)

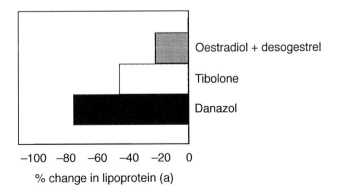

Figure 10. Effects of androgenic compounds on lipoprotein (a). (Adapted from Crook et al, 1992b; Rymer et al, 1993; Marsh et al, 1994.)

  Depending on their androgenicity, progestogens reduce VLDL secretion
and this results in a lowering of triglycerides (Crook et al, 1992a), an effect
which is clearly beneficial. Such an effect is not seen with the non-
androgenic progestogens. The duration of progestogen administration in
HRT may also be important. For example, desogestrel is a progestogen
derived from norgestrel and has less androgenic effects than the parent
molecule. However, continuous administration of desogestrel together with
oestradiol results in a lowering of HDL_2 by 26% (Marsh et al, 1994)
compared with a reduction of only 10% during the combined phase of
continuous conjugated equine oestrogens but cyclical norgestrel (Crook et
al, 1992a).

  Depending on the choice of steroids used and their route of administration, it is possible to obtain a variety of different effects on lipids and
lipoproteins with HRT. Overall, the effects of most HRT on lipids and
lipoproteins would seem in balance to be beneficial, and of course there are
many other non-lipid risk factors which are also beneficially affected by
HRT (Stevenson et al, 1994).

BODY FAT DISTRIBUTION

There is an association between the distribution of body fat and CHD
which is independent of obesity itself. This may be of importance since
it is the abdominal (android) fat which has been associated with an
increased risk of CHD whereas the lower body segment (gynoid) fat does
not appear to be related to any increased risk. The android fat distribution
is typical of the male whereas the gynoid fat distribution, particularly
around the hips, thighs and buttocks, is typical of the female. In our
preliminary studies of 40 post-menopausal women, we found that android
fat mass correlated negatively with HDL and HDL_2 cholesterol concentrations and positively with triglycerides (Stevenson et al, 1990). In a
study of over 100 healthy men, we again found that android fat rather
than overall adiposity was associated with adverse metabolic changes
such as lower HDL_2 cholesterol, higher triglycerides, and increased
insulin resistance (Walton et al, 1995), and hence with an increased CHD
risk. In a further study of non-obese men with CHD, higher proportions
of android fat were observed than healthy matched controls (Ley et al,
1994). It therefore seems reasonable to assume that android obesity is
also a CHD risk factor for women. Loss of ovarian hormones at the
menopause results in a redistribution of body fat towards the male pattern
with a relative increase in the proportion of android fat and a relative
decrease in the proportion of fat in the female gynoid distribution (Ley
et al, 1992). This redistribution of body fat would therefore be expected
to be associated with an increase in CHD risk. HRT does not normally
cause a significant increase in weight, and may actually improve the
distribution of body fat by limiting or reversing increases in the android
distribution.

COAGULATION AND FIBRINOLYSIS

The haemostatic system is a dynamic system which is designed to provide immediate clot formation at the site of haemorrhage whilst at the same time preventing intravascular clot formation. This is achieved by balances between coagulation and fibrinolysis which are in turn achieved by complex interplays between pro-thrombotic and anti-thrombotic factors and pro-fibrinolytic and anti-fibrinolytic factors.

Changes in haemostatic factors may be linked with the insulin resistance syndrome. Increased insulin concentrations are linked with increased levels of PAI-1, and increased PAI-1 levels have been associated with CHD. The effects of the menopause on these have not been studied widely and it is often difficult to separate these effects from those of ageing. Factor VII is increased in post-menopausal women (Bonithon-Kopp et al, 1990) as is fibrinogen (Bonithon-Kopp et al, 1990; Meade et al, 1990), although ageing has a marked effect on the latter. Ageing also increases protein C and antithrombin III (Meade et al, 1990) but it is not established whether the menopause has an effect (Pinto et al, 1990). Despite these changes in pro-thrombotic and anti-thrombotic factors, there does not appear to be any menopausal effect on reaction products of thrombin activity (Pinto et al, 1990). With regard to fibrinolysis, tissue plasminogen activator (tPA) increases with age (Rånby et al, 1986) but PAI-1 concentrations are also higher following menopause (Heinrich et al, 1991). These findings taken together lead to the conclusion that there is a reduction in fibrinolytic activity following the menopause but no reduction, or even an increase, in coagulant activity. Thus the balance between coagulation and fibrinolysis is tipped towards the former.

The effects of HRT on haemostasis are somewhat complex (Winkler, 1992), but overall the effect appears to favour fibrinolysis rather than coagulation. This is compatible with the fact that HRT does not consistently cause an increase in venous thromboembolism (Lowe et al, 1992) and indeed reduces the incidence of arterial thromboembolism (Paganini-Hill et al, 1988). A recent detailed study has shown no significant change in any haemostatic parameter with transdermal oestradiol (Fox et al, 1993). No data are available on HRT effects in patients with coagulopathies, but it seems likely that the use of transdermal oestradiol would be advisable, irrespective of the progestogen used, should such patients require HRT.

DIRECT ARTERIAL EFFECTS

This topic will be dealt with in detail in another chapter, but direct arterial effects are another important way in which HRT produces its benefits on the cardiovascular system. In post-menopausal women, the menopause results in an increase in arterial waveform pulsatility index, an index reflecting reduced arterial compliance, in the carotid artery during the first few years

(Gangar et al, 1991). The administration of oestradiol-17β reverses this increase (Gangar et al, 1991), and this effect is not abolished by progestogen administration (Hillard et al, 1992).

The action of oestradiol on the artery is mediated through endothelium-dependent mechanisms, calcium-dependent mechanisms, and other mechanisms such as angiotensin-1-converting enzyme reduction (Proudler et al, 1995). It is also conceivable that some of the metabolic changes induced by oestrogen administration may themselves have arterial effects. For example, in post-menopausal women with syndrome X we have found that insulin resistance correlates with the response of their ECG exercise test ischaemic change to oestradiol administration (Godsland et al, 1994).

SUMMARY

There is little doubt that the metabolic disturbances seen following the loss of ovarian function are most important in the development of cardio-vascular disease in women. The loss of hormones at the menopause appears to reduce both insulin secretion and elimination, but increasing insulin resistance thereafter brings about an increase in circulating insulin concentrations. Changes in lipids and lipoproteins are in an adverse direction, as are changes in body fat distribution, and changes in haemostatic factors would tend to favour coagulation rather than fibrinolysis.

HRT with oestrogen appears to improve most of the metabolic abnormalities related to the menopause, but this is in part dependent on the type of oestrogen used and the route of administration. The addition of progestogen may influence the metabolic changes induced by oestrogens, and this will vary according to the type of the progestogen. Overall, the metabolic effects of any of the current HRT regimens would seem likely to be beneficial for CHD. Nevertheless, future HRT regimens should ideally be tailored to produce the most favourable changes in CHD metabolic risk factors, particularly in the case of the regimens which attempt to avoid cyclical bleeding.

REFERENCES

Abbott W, Lillioja S & Young A (1987) Relationships between plasma lipoprotein concentrations and insulin action in an obese hyperinsulinaemic population. *Diabetes* **36:** 897–904.

Austin MA, Breslow JL, Hennekens CH et al (1988) Low density lipoprotein subclass patterns and risk of myocardial infarction. *Journal of the American Medical Association* **26:** 1917–1921.

Båvenholm P, Proudler AJ, Tornvall P et al (1995) Insulin, intact and split proinsulin and coronary artery disease in young men. *Circulation* **92:** 1422–1429.

Bengtsson C, Björkelund C, Lapidus L & Lissner L (1993) Associations of serum lipid concentrations and obesity with mortality in women: 20 year follow up of participants in prospective population study in Gothenburg, Sweden. *British Medical Journal* **307:** 1385–1388.

Bonithon-Kopp C, Scarabin P-Y, Darne B et al (1990) Menopause-related changes in lipids and lipoproteins and some other cardiovascular risk factors. *International Journal of Epidemiology* **19:** 42–48.

Cagnacci A, Soldani R, Carriero PL et al (1992) Effects of low doses of transdermal 17β-estradiol on carbohydrate metabolism in postmenopausal women. *Journal of Clinical Endocrinology and Metabolism* **74:** 1396–1400.

Campos H, McNamara JR, Wilson PWF et al (1988) Differences in low density lipoprotein subfractions and apolipoproteins in premenopausal and postmenopausal women. *Journal of Clinical Endocrinology and Metabolism* **67:** 30–35.

Campos H, Sacks FM, Walsh BW et al (1993) Differential effects of estrogen on low-density lipoprotein subclasses in healthy postmenopausal women. *Metabolism* **42:** 1153–1158.

Crook D, Cust MP, Gangar KF et al (1992a) Comparison of transdermal and oral estrogen/progestin hormone replacement therapy: effects on serum lipids and lipoproteins. *American Journal of Obstetrics and Gynecology* **166:** 950–955.

Crook D, Sidhu M, Seed M et al (1992b) Lipoprotein Lp(a) levels are reduced by danazol, an anabolic steroid. *Atherosclerosis* **92:** 41–47.

Dahlén G, Ericson C & Berg K (1978) In vitro studies of the interaction of isolated Lp(a) lipoprotein and other serum lipoproteins with glycosaminoglycans. *Clinical Genetics* **14:** 36–42.

Donahue RP, Abbott RD, Reed DM & Katsuhiko Y (1987) Post-challenge glucose concentration and coronary heart disease in men of Japanese ancestry. *Diabetes* **36:** 689–692.

Farrish E, Rolton HA, Barnes JF & Hart DM (1991) Lipoprotein (a) concentrations in postmenopausal women taking norethisterone. *British Medical Journal* **303:** 694.

Ferrannini E, Buzziogli G, Bonadonna R et al (1987) Insulin resistance in essential hypertension. *New England Journal of Medicine* **317:** 350–357.

Fox J, George AJ, Newton JR et al (1993) Effect of transdermal oestradiol on the haemostatic balance of menopausal women. *Maturitas* **18:** 55–64.

Freis JF, Green IW & Levine S (1989) Health promotion and the compression of morbidity. *Lancet* i: 481–483.

Fuller JH, Shipley MJ, Rose G et al (1983) Mortality from coronary heart disease and stroke in relation to degree of glycaemia: the Whitehall Study. *British Medical Journal* **287:** 867–870.

Gangar KF, Vyas S, Whitehead M et al (1991) Pulsatility index in internal carotid artery in relation to transdermal oestradiol and time since menopause. *Lancet* **338:** 839–842.

Godsland IF, Gangar KF, Walton C et al (1993) Insulin resistance, secretion, and elimination in postmenopausal women receiving oral or transdermal hormone replacement therapy. *Metabolism* **42:** 846–853.

Godsland IF, Rosano GMC, Proudler AJ et al. (1994) Insulin resistance in postmenopausal women with syndrome X who do not respond to estrogen therapy. *Circulation* **90:** I-554.

Godsland IF, Crook D, Stevenson JC et al (1995) Insulin resistance syndrome in postmenopausal women with cardiological syndrome X. *British Heart Journal* **74:** 47–52.

Gordon T, Kannel WB, Hjortland MC & McNamara PM. (1978) Menopause and coronary heart disease. The Framingham Study. *Annals of Internal Medicine* **89:** 157–161.

Heinrich J, Sandkamp M, Kokott R et al (1991) Relationship of lipoprotein (a) to variables of coagulation and fibrinolysis in a healthy population. *Clinical Chemistry* **37:** 1950–1954.

Hillard TC, Bourne TH, Whitehead MI et al (1992) Differential effects of transdermal estradiol and sequential progestogens on impedance to flow within the uterine arteries of postmenopausal women. *Fertility and Sterility* **58:** 959–963.

Jarnet RJ, McCartney P & Keen H (1982) The Bedford Survey: ten year mortality rates in newly diagnosed diabetics and normoglycaemic controls and risk for coronary heart disease in borderline diabetics. *Diabetologia* **22:** 79–84.

Jensen J, Nilas L & Christiansen C (1990) Influence of menopause on serum lipids and lipoproteins. *Maturitas* **12:** 321.

Juhan-Vague I, Alessi MC, Joly P et al (1989) Plasma plasminogen activator inhibitor 1 in angina pectoris. Influence of plasma insulin and acute-phase response. *Arteriosclerosis* **9:** 362–367.

Kannel WB (1982) Meaning of a downward trend in cardiovascular mortality. *Journal of the American Medical Association* **247:** 877–880.

Kemp HG, Vokonas PS, Cohn PF & Gorlin R (1973) The anginal syndrome associated with normal coronary arteriograms. Report of a six year experience. *American Journal of Medicine* **54:** 735–752.

Krauss RM (1991) The tangled web of coronary risk factors. *American Journal of Medicine* **90 (supplement 2A):** 36–41.

Kuller LH, Gutai JP, Meilahn E et al (1990) Relationship of endogenous sex steroid hormones to lipids and apoproteins in postmenopausal women. *Arteriosclerosis* **10:** 1058.

LaCroix AZ, Haynes SG, Savage DD & Havlik RJ (1989) Rose questionnaire angina among United States black, white and Mexican–American women and men. *American Journal of Epidemiology* **129:** 669–686.

Ley CJ, Lees B & Stevenson JC (1992) Sex- and menopause-associated changes in body-fat distribution. *American Journal of Clinical Nutrition* **55:** 950–954.

Ley CJ, Swan J, Godsland IF et al (1994) Insulin resistance, lipoproteins, body fat and hemostasis in non-obese males with angina and normal or abnormal coronary angiograms. *Journal of the American College of Cardiologists* **23:** 377–383.

Loscalzo J, Weinfeld M, Fless GM & Scanu AM (1990) Lipoprotein (a), fibrin binding and plasminogen activation. *Arteriosclerosis* **10:** 240–245.

Lowe GDO, Greer IA, Cooke TG et al (1992) Risk of and prophylaxis for venous thromboembolism in hospital patients. *British Medical Journal* **305:** 567–574.

Mahrabian M, Qiao J-H, Hyman R et al (1993) Influence of the apoA-II gene locus on HDL levels and fatty streak development in mice. *Arteriosclerosis and Thrombosis* **13:** 1–10.

Marsh MS, Crook D, Whitcroft SIJ et al (1994) Effect of continuous combined estrogen and desogestrel replacement therapy on serum lipids and lipoproteins. *Obstetrics and Gynecology* **83:** 19–23.

Matthews KA, Meilahn E, Kuller LH et al (1989) Menopause and risk factors for coronary heart disease. *New England Journal of Medicine* **321:** 641–646.

Meade TW, Dyer S, Howart DJ et al (1990) Antithrombin III and procoagulant activity: sex differences and effect of the menopause. *British Journal of Haematology* **74:** 77–81.

Meilahn EN, Kuller LH, Matthews KA & Stein A (1991) Lp(a) concentrations among pre- and postmenopausal women over time: the Healthy Women Study. *Circulation* **84 (supplement II):** 546.

Miller NE (1987) Associations of high-density lipoprotein subclasses and apolipoproteins with ischaemic heart disease and coronary atherosclerosis. *American Heart Journal* **113:** 589–597.

Notelovitz M, Johnston M, Smith S & Kitchens C (1987) Metabolic and hormonal effects of 25 mg and 50 mg 17β estradiol implants in surgically menopausal women. *Obstetrics and Gynecology* **70:** 749–754.

Oliver MF & Boyd GS (1959) Effect of bilateral ovariectomy on coronary artery disease and serum lipid levels. *Lancet* **ii:** 690–692.

Paganini-Hill A, Ross RK & Henderson BE (1988) Postmenopausal oestrogen treatment and stroke: a prospective study. *British Medical Journal* **297:** 519–522.

Pinto S, Rostagno C, Coppo M et al. (1990) No sign of increased thrombin generation in menopause. *Thrombosis Research* **58:** 645–651.

Proudler AJ, Felton CV & Stevenson JC (1992) Ageing and the response of plasma insulin, glucose and C-peptide concentrations to intravenous glucose in postmenopausal women. *Clinical Science* **83:** 489–494.

Proudler AJ, Ahmed AIH, Crook D et al (1995) Hormone replacement therapy and serum angiotensin-converting-enzyme activity in postmenopausal women. *Lancet* **346:** 89–90.

Rånby M, Bergsdorf N, Nilsson T et al (1986) Age dependence of tissue plasminogen activator concentrations in plasma as studied by an improved enzyme-linked immunosorbent assay. *Clinical Chemistry* **32:** 2160–2165.

Reaven GM (1988) Role of insulin resistance in human disease. *Diabetes* **37:** 1595–1607.

Reaven GM, Ida Chen Y-D, Jeppesen J et al (1993) Insulin resistance and hyperinsulinaemia in individuals with small dense low density lipoprotein particles. *Journal of Clinical Investigation* **92:** 141–146.

Rönnemaa T, Laakso M, Pyörälä K et al (1991) High fasting plasma insulin is an indicator of coronary heart disease in non-insulin-dependent diabetic patients and non-diabetic subjects. *Arteriosclerosis* **11:** 80–90.

Rubin EM, Krauss R, Spangler E et al (1991) Inhibition of early atherogenesis in transgenic mice by human apolipoprotein A-I. *Nature* **353:** 265–267.

Rymer J, Crook D, Sidhu M et al (1993) Effects of tibolone on serum concentrations of lipoprotein (a) in postmenopausal women. *Acta Endocrinologica* **128:** 259–262.

Sack MN, Rader DJ & Cannon RO (1994) Oestrogen and inhibition of oxidation of low-density lipoproteins in postmenopausal women. *Lancet* **343:** 269–270.

Shen MMS, Krauss RM, Lindgren FT & Forte TM (1981) Heterogeneity of serum low density lipoproteins in normal human subjects. *Journal of Lipid Research* **22:** 236–244.

Spellacy WN, Buhi WC & Birk SA (1972) The effects of estrogens on carbohydrate metabolism:

glucose, insulin and growth hormone studies on one hundred and seventy one women ingesting Premarin, mestranol and ethinyl estradiol for six months. *American Journal of Obstetrics and Gynecology* **114:** 378–392.

Stevenson JC (1995) The metabolic and cardiovascular consequences of HRT. *British Journal of Clinical Practice* **49:** 87–90.

Stevenson JC, Lees B, Bruce R et al (1990) Influence of body composition on lipid metabolism in postmenopausal women. In Christiansen C & Overgaard K (eds) *Osteoporosis*, pp 1837–1838. Copenhagen: Osteopress ApS.

Stevenson JC, Crook D & Godsland IF (1993) Influence of age and menopause on serum lipids and lipoproteins in healthy women. *Atherosclerosis* **98:** 83–90.

Stevenson JC, Crook D, Godsland IF et al (1994) Hormone replacement therapy and the cardiovascular system. Nonlipid effects. *Drugs,* **47 (supplement 2):** 35–41.

Stout R (1990) Insulin and atheroma: 20-yr perspective: *Diabetes Care* **13:** 631–654.

Swan JW, Walton C, Godsland IF et al (1994) The insulin resistance syndrome as a feature of cardiological syndrome X in non-obese men. *British Heart Journal* **71:** 41–44.

Sznajderman M & Oliver MF (1963) Spontaneous premature menopause, ischaemic heart disease and serum lipids. *Lancet* **i:** 962–964.

Tikkanen MJ, Kuusi T, Vartiainen E & Nikkila EA (1979) Treatment of post-menopausal hypercholesterolaemia with oestradiol. *Acta Obstetrica et Gynecologica* **88 (supplement):** 83–88.

Tribble DL, Holl LG, Wood PD & Krauss RM (1992) Variations in oxidative susceptibility among six low density lipoprotein subfractions of differing density and particle size. *Atherosclerosis* **93:** 189–199.

Utermann G (1989) The mysteries of lipoprotein (a). *Science* **264:** 904–910.

van der Mooren MJ, de Graaf J, Demacker PN et al (1994) Changes in the low-density lipoprotein profile during 17 beta-oestradiol-dydrogesterone therapy in postmenopausal women. *Metabolism* **43:** 799–802.

Walton C, Godsland IF, Proudler AJ et al (1993) The effects of the menopause on insulin sensitivity, secretion and elimination in non-obese, healthy women. *European Journal of Clinical Investigation* **23:** 466–473.

Walton C, Lees B, Godsland IF, Crook D & Stevenson JC (1995) Relationship between insulin metabolism, serum lipid profile, body fat distribution and blood pressure in healthy men. *Atherosclerosis* **118:** 35–43.

Warden CH, Hedrick CC, Qiao J-H et al (1993) Atherosclerosis in transgenic mice overexpressing apolipoprotein AII. *Science* **261:** 469–471.

Welborn TA & Wearne K (1979) Coronary heart disease incidence and cardiovascular mortality in Busselton with reference to glucose and insulin concentrations. *Diabetes Care* **2:** 154–160.

Westerveld HT, Kock LAW, van Rijn JM et al (1995) 17β-estradiol improves postprandial lipid metabolism in postmenopausal women. *Journal of Clinical Endocrinology and Metabolism* **80:** 249–253.

Whitcroft SI, Crook D, Marsh MS et al (1994) Long-term effects of oral and transdermal hormone replacement therapies on serum lipid and lipoprotein concentrations. *Obstetrics and Gynecology* **84:** 222–226.

Wilhelmsen L, Bengtsson C, Elmfeldt D et al (1977) Multiple risk prediction of myocardial infarction in women as compared with men. *British Heart Journal* **39:** 1179–1185.

Williams KJ & Tabas I (1995) The response-to-retention hypothesis of early atherogenesis. *Arteriosclerosis and Thrombosis* **15:** 551–561.

Winkler UH (1992) Menopause, hormone replacement therapy and cardiovascular disease: a review of haemostaseological findings. *Fibrinolysis* **6 (supplement 3):** 5–10.

Witteman JCM, Grobbee DE, Kok FJ et al (1989) Increased risk of atherosclerosis in women after the menopause. *British Medical Journal* **298:** 642–644.

Wolfe BM & Huff MW (1993) Effect of low dosage progestin-only administration upon plasma triglycerides and lipoprotein metabolism in postmenopausal women. *Journal of Clinical Investigation* **92:** 456–461.

Yashiro A, O'Neil J & Hoff HF (1993) Insoluble complex formation of lipoprotein (a) with low density lipoprotein in the presence of calcium ions. *Journal of Biological Chemistry* **268:** 4709–4715.

8

The menopause and the skeleton: key issues

JOHN A. KANIS

Osteoporosis and fractures occur much more frequently in women than men. For white women aged 50 years, the remaining life-time risk of an osteoporotic fracture lies between 30 and 40%, threefold higher than that in men (WHO, 1994). There are several reasons for the high prevalence of fractures in women. First, women have a lower skeletal mass at maturity compared to men. Second, although bone loss occurs in both men and women with age, the loss is substantially greater in women. Third, life expectancy is greater in women than in men, and they are, therefore, exposed for longer to a given risk. Finally, in the elderly, women seem to fall more frequently than men for reasons which have yet to be determined. Therefore, much attention has been focused on the causes and management of osteoporosis in women, and particularly on the use of hormone replacement therapy (HRT) at the time of the menopause.

There is good evidence for a causal relationship between the menopause and post-menopausal osteoporosis. Bone loss coincides with gonadal deficiency and this can be prevented by the administration of gonadal steroids. Despite the wealth of evidence, there are still uncertainties concerning the activity of oestrogens and progestogens on bone and the manner in which these agents should be used in preventive strategies for osteoporosis.

MECHANISMS OF BONE LOSS AT THE MENOPAUSE

The manner in which bone loss occurs in post-menopausal osteoporosis is determined by changes in skeletal metabolism and architecture. The skeleton is comprised of compact and cancellous (trabecular) bone. In the healthy adult at maturity, bone mass is neither increasing nor decreasing, but there is a considerable turnover of bone, of which 95% or more is accounted for by remodelling. The remodelling process comprises a discrete series of cellular events on bone surfaces. The surface of cancellous bone available for remodelling is much greater than that of cortical bone, despite cancellous bone occupying a minority of the total skeletal mass. Because of the high surface to volume ratio of cancellous bone, osteoporosis commonly affects cancellous sites earlier and more floridly than cortical sites. This may explain, in part, the occurrence of vertebral fractures early in the natural history of osteoporosis, whereas hip fractures are a much later event.

At the start of bone remodelling, osteoclasts assemble or differentiate together to excavate an erosion cavity on the bone surface (Figure 1). Once erosion is complete, the osteoclasts or bone resorbing cells disappear and are replaced by osteoblasts which are attracted principally to the sites of previous resorption and in-fill the erosion cavity with new bone. Remodelling confers greater strength to bone in vivo than suggested by the properties of bone in vitro, since the process allows the removal and repair of fatigue damage.

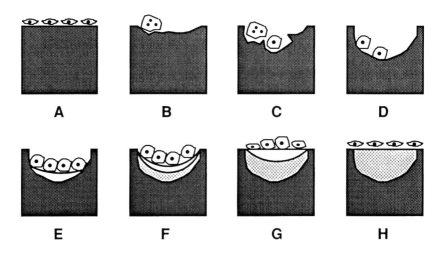

Figure 1. Steps in the bone remodelling sequence of cancellous bone. Early in the remodelling sequence, osteoclasts are attracted to quiescent bone surfaces (A), and excavate a resorption cavity (B,C). Mononuclear cells smooth off the resorption cavity (D), which is a subsequent site for the attraction of osteoblasts which synthesize an osteoid matrix (E). Continuous new matrix synthesis (F) is followed by calcification (G) of the newly formed bone. When complete, lining cells once more overlie the trabecular surface (H).

In health there are several million active remodelling sites in the skeleton, but these occupy a minority of the bone surface (15 to 20%). One of the early effects of gonadal deficiency is to accelerate the rate of bone turnover. All the elements of turnover—resorption, formation and mineralisation—are accelerated due to an increase in the generation or activation of new bone remodelling units on the bone surface. The earliest effect is therefore an increased number of osteoclasts since resorption precedes formation in the remodelling sequence. There is still no clear understanding of the way in which oestrogens affect osteoclast metabolism and oestrogen receptors, in low density, have only been identified on osteoblasts.

Since the number of bone remodelling units is increased, then at any one time a progressively greater surface of bone will be occupied by remodelling events. Since the process of bone remodelling implies a net deficit of bone (until resorption cavities are completely in-filled), the skeletal volume missing at any one time will increase proportionately according to the number of functional bone remodelling units (Kanis, 1991; Figure 2). A fivefold increase in bone turnover would decrease the mineral content of cancellous bone by more than 20% under steady state conditions, cortical bone by more than 3% and total body mineral content by more than 7%. Because of the prolonged turnover time of the skeleton, it may take several years to reach a new steady state where skeletal mass is no longer decreasing. This accounts in part for the accelerated bone losses that occur in the early years after the menopause.

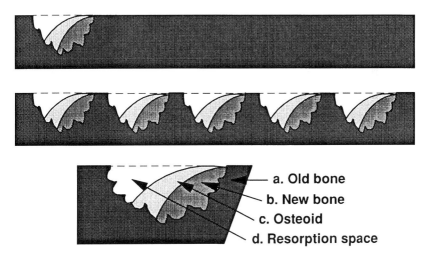

a. Old bone
b. New bone
c. Osteoid
d. Resorption space

Figure 2. Effect of skeletal turnover on bone and calcium balance. The upper panel is a schematic representation of a bony trabeculum showing normal remodelling activity occurring on 15% of the bone surface. The resorption space (d) occupies 2% of the bone volume, and a somewhat smaller amount is occupied by osteoid (c. 1.5%) accounting for 3.5% of cancellous bone volume. When turnover is increased fivefold, without affecting the balance between resorption and formation, the resorption and osteoid space is increased to 17% of bone volume. In addition, new bone formed at each site is not completely mineralised (b), increasing the mineral deficit, so that the apparent mineral density is increased by 20%.

In addition, bone loss in post-menopausal osteoporosis also arises due to an imbalance between the amount of mineral and matrix removed and that subsequently incorporated into each erosion cavity (Eriksen, 1986), so that skeletal mass decreases incrementally with each remodelling event. When bone turnover is also accelerated, this amplifies the rate of bone loss (Figure 3). Conversely, a decrease in turnover will decrease the rate of bone loss, even when the balance between formation and resorption and each remodelling site is unaffected. Thus, oestrogen deficiency increases bone turnover and induces an imbalance between resorption and formation, and thereby accelerates skeletal losses.

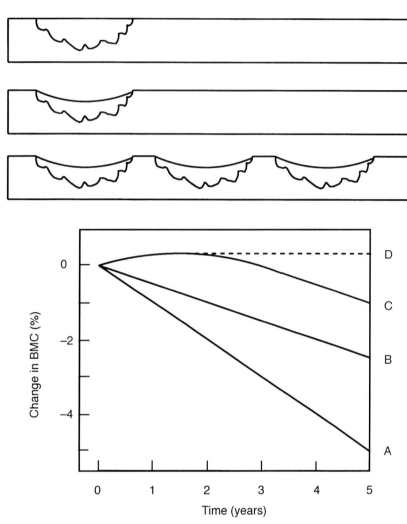

Figure 3. The upper panel shows a schematic representation of cancellous bone surfaces to illustrate the effect of balance and remodelling on the rate of bone loss. The upper trabeculum shows the in-filling of a resorption bay with an equal volume of new bone. In hypogonadism, less bone is deposited in resorption cavities (centre). If bone turnover is increased without altering this balance (lower), the rate of cancellous bone loss will increase in proportion to the increment in bone turnover. The lower panel shows the expected effects of decreasing bone turnover in osteoporosis. The relationship between bone mineral content (BMC) with time is shown for a patient losing 1% of bone mass per year due to an imbalance of bone at remodelling sites (A). If bone turnover is halved without altering the imbalance between the amounts formed and resorbed, the rate of bone loss is halved (B). The administration of an inhibitor of bone resorption permits continued formation at pre-existing erosion sites, so that BMC increases to fill this resorption space. When bone formation decreases to match the prevailing rate of bone resorption, bone loss will occur once more, albeit at a slower rate than before treatment (C). Agents that additionally adjust the imbalance between resorption and formation are expected to show an increment in bone mass over two years which is thereafter sustained (D).

EFFECT OF OESTROGENS ON BONE

A logical intervention in the prevention of osteoporosis is the use of gonadal steroids (oestrogens and progestogens). Other preventive agents include the calcitonins, pharmacological doses of calcium, the bisphosphonates and, in some countries, vitamin D. All these decrease the rate of bone remodelling and thereby the rate of bone loss. It is important to recognize that many of these agents have a primary effect to inhibit bone resorption by limiting the accession of osteoclasts to bone to create new erosion cavities. After the onset of treatment, in-filling of existing erosion cavities will continue so that skeletal mass may increase transiently for several years until a new steady state is achieved (Figure 3). This non-linear pattern of response has been well documented for all inhibitors of bone turnover and is important to recognize when assessing the long-term effects of intervention. The relatively small increments in skeletal mass after a year or so of treatment should not be interpreted as an anabolic response in the sense that the increment does not continue indefinitely, and even if given for long enough the treatment would not restore skeletal mass in patients with established osteoporosis.

Agents such as pharmacological amounts of calcium and calcitonin appear to induce transient increments in skeletal mass over a year or two of treatment. Thereafter bone loss occurs, albeit at a rate slower than in untreated patients (Figure 3). This suggests that these agents decrease bone turnover, but do not correct the imbalance between the amount of bone resorbed and that formed at each remodelling site. A great deal of evidence indicates that the gonadal steroids, particularly oestrogens and the androgenic progestogens, induce small increments in skeletal mass which are not followed by a progressive decrease in bone density. Thus, oestrogens in appropriate doses prevent bone loss, irrespective of whether they are given in the immediate peri-menopausal period or when bone loss is established (Lindsay, 1990). This is because oestrogens not only decrease the rate of bone turnover, a property shared by other inhibitors of bone turnover, but may also correct the imbalance at each remodelling site.

Few dose response studies have been undertaken to assess the long-term effects of oestrogens on skeletal balance. In the case of conjugated oestrogens, 0.625 mg daily is the average dose that spares bone losses at the appendicular skeleton (Lindsay et al, 1984). What is not known is whether supraphysiological doses of oestrogens have added effects on skeletal mass; there is evidence for and against this, although it is inadequate to make a sound judgement (Garnett et al, 1990). Against this background it has been difficult to assess the effects, if any, on skeletal balance of adding progestogens to oestrogens. Current evidence would suggest that C19 derivatives such as norethisterone do have skeletal effects which might be additive (Christiansen et al, 1985), but these agents also have anabolic and oestrogenic activity; the effects of C21 derivatives such as medroxyprogesterone are less certain (Grey et al, 1996).

OSTEOPOROSIS AND ITS CONSEQUENCES

The currently accepted definition of osteoporosis is 'a disease characterized by low bone mass and microarchitectural deterioration of bone tissue leading to enhanced bone fragility and a consequent increase in fracture risk' (Anonymous, 1993). There are now several techniques which accurately measure bone mass at regional sites, and these provide a frame-work for the diagnosis of osteoporosis. These include single and dual energy X-ray absorptiometry which measure bone mineral content or apparent bone mineral density (BMD), these techniques form the basis for the definition of osteoporosis and provide a cut-off for BMD that identifies most women with osteoporotic fractures. Bone mass measurements are also taken to assess the future risk of fracture, so that more than one cut-off is appropriate.

Four general diagnostic categories have been established in women (WHO, 1994).

1. *Normal.* A value for BMD or bone mineral content that is within 1 SD of the young adult mean.
2. *Low bone mass (osteopenia).* A value for BMD or bone mineral content more than 1 SD below the young adult mean, but less than 2.5 SD below this value.
3. *Osteoporosis.* A value for BMD or bone mineral content 2.5 SD or more below the young adult mean.
4. *Severe osteoporosis (established osteoporosis).* A value for BMD or bone mineral content more than 2.5 SD below the young adult mean in the presence of one or more fragility fractures.

Because the distribution of bone mass in the female population is normal, the proportion of women affected by osteoporosis at one site increases markedly with age, coincident with the loss of bone that occurs at the menopause. By the age of 70 years, more than a third of women will have osteoporosis of the femoral neck (Kanis et al, 1994). Osteoporosis of the hip will affect 20% of post-menopausal women comparable to the life-time risk of a single osteoporotic fracture such as of the hip.

Classical fractures associated with osteoporosis include vertebral crush fractures, fractures of the distal forearm and hip fracture. The osteo-porotic skeleton is, however, more liable to fracture at many other sites. Because bone density decreases progressively with age, the incidence of osteoporosis increases in an exponential manner. The incidence of many osteoporotic fractures also increases exponentially in both men and women.

Of the various osteoporotic fractures, that of the hip carries the greatest morbidity, some mortality and socio-economic costs. For example, direct hospital costs for fractures, in England and Wales amount to £220 million, of which nearly 90% are accounted for by hip fracture. Because hip fracture invariably requires hospitalization, more is known about the consequences of this fracture than for vertebral or Colles fractures (WHO, 1994).

EFFECTS OF HRT ON FRACTURES

A wealth of data from prospective studies indicate that the use of HRT will prevent bone loss at the menopause and thereafter (Lindsay, 1990). In some women, the doses required to prevent bone loss are higher than those required to treat menopausal symptoms, but provided that the dose is adequate, the oestrogens will prevent bone loss more or less completely, irrespective of when, in the course of osteoporotic bone loss, they are given. On the assumption that bone loss resumes at the expected rate when treatment is stopped, the effects of HRT on fracture rates would be marked. Thus, HRT taken for 10 years following the menopause would defer the risk of fracture with age by 10 years. Calculations based on this premise suggest that the risk of hip fracture would be reduced by more than 50%, and epidemiological data support this view (WHO, 1994).

Case control and cohort studies consistently report that HRT reduces the risk of hip fracture in perimenopausal and post-menopausal women. In addition, randomized prospective studies show a decrease in vertebral fracture frequency of greater than 50% (Lufkin et al, 1992). The pooled estimate of the relative risk of hip fracture comparing oestrogen users with non-users is 0.7 (95% confidence interval, 0.6 to 0.8), and there is some evidence that the risk of hip fracture decreases with increasing duration of oestrogen use (WHO, 1994). The androgenic progestogens also prevent bone loss, and several studies have found that the combined use of oestrogen and a variety of progestogen regimens also achieve this. These data suggest that progestogens do not adversely influence the effects of oestrogens on fractures due to osteoporosis.

All these observations have lent credence to the view that an optimal prevention strategy for osteoporosis lies in the widespread use of HRT in women. The logical time for such intervention is at the menopause, which clearly signals an oestrogen deficient state. Furthermore, most therapeutic interventions, including HRT, do not substantially increase bone mass; rather they prevent further losses, suggesting that early rather than later intervention is preferable (Kanis, 1991). In addition, progressive bone loss is associated with the discontinuity of trabecular elements in cancellous bone, particularly in hypogonadal states (Parfitt, 1984). These trabecular discontinuities decrease the mechanical competence of bone out of pro-portion to the amount of bone lost. Moreover, once trabecular perforation has occurred, there is good evidence to suggest that the remnant structures atrophy, perhaps due to a change in the stresses applied through cancellous bone. Because bone remodelling is a surface based event, the atrophy of remnant structures means that interventions that act by influencing bone remodelling are at best capable of thickening trabecular elements but are unlikely to increase trabecular numbers to normal (Kanis, 1984).

Although there is a convincing causal relationship between oestrogen deficiency and osteoporotic fracture, there are a number of considerations which suggest that attention has focused too much on gonadal deficiency as a cause of osteoporosis, and that HRT given at the menopause may not be the most logical approach to its management.

USE AND TARGETTING OF HRT

A first consideration is the difficulty in targetting HRT at the time of the menopause. The issues of HRT are much wider than those of osteoporosis alone; additional benefits include a decrease in cardiovascular-related morbidity and mortality, and the control of post-menopausal symptoms. The risks from opposed regimens relate largely to whether the risks for breast cancer are increased. Where the risks and benefits of HRT are compared, the benefits of a decrease in cardiovascular disease are very much greater than those of a decreased incidence of osteoporotic fracture. If the risk of breast cancer is increased, this is small; notwithstanding, any increase in risk of a common disease has major implications and this could nullify any gains from antifracture efficacy. For these reasons many now consider that the targetting of HRT to women at risk from osteoporosis at the menopause is not justified, at least in a screening programme. It seems illogical to target HRT on the basis of BMD, where the major benefits and risks are extraskeletal (WHO, 1994). Rather, HRT might be more optimally used in individuals with a high risk of cardiovascular disease and avoided in those where the risk of breast cancer is high. Unfortunately, identification of these 'at risk' groups at the time of the menopause is difficult. These considerations should not be interpreted to mean that assessments of BMD are not indicated in certain 'at risk' groups, for example, women with a premature menopause. They do, however, suggest that the case for wide-spread screening of BMD at the time of the menopause is inappropriate, because giving HRT widely is for other reasons.

A further problem with the use of HRT is that the uptake in many countries is relatively low. Moreover, it is accepted that for significant skeletal benefit, HRT should be given continuously for five to 10 years. Even in countries where the uptake of HRT is high, long-term compliance is low, largely because the major advantage perceived by post-menopausal women is the alleviation of post-menopausal symptoms; this is achieved by treatment for several months rather than several years.

These practical considerations suggest that there is much to be learnt about the reasons for poor compliance and a need to develop new strategies for HRT. In addition, the identification of significant risk factors for breast cancer and cardiovascular disease is a necessary prerequisite for the more generalized use of HRT.

EFFICACY OF HRT

There is good evidence that HRT can prevent bone loss in the vast majority of women during a 10-year course of treatment (Lindsay, 1990). Current evidence would suggest that HRT should not be given for longer than 10 years. More prolonged experience with these agents may modify these recommendations in time but, from a practical point of view, treatment for life is currently not envisaged. A crucial consideration relates, therefore, not to the efficacy of therapeutic intervention during the course of treatment, but more to the offset of therapeutic effects when HRT is stopped. Some observational studies have suggested that the effects of oestrogen on hip fractures are less in elderly women than at the time of the menopause (Law et al, 1991). It has been argued that when oestrogens are stopped, catch-up bone loss occurs so that 10 to 20 years or so thereafter, bone mass in treated patients would be the same as in untreated controls (Kanis, 1995; Figure 4). This argument is not, however, perfect, since the increased mortality of patients with osteoporosis decreases the apparent efficacy computed from retrospective epidemiological studies. Thus, the evaluation of relative risk for hip fractures in untreated versus treated women may be underestimated in the elderly because of the selective loss of untreated osteoporotic patients (Kanis and Stevenson, 1994). Indeed, prospective studies suggest that oestrogen withdrawal does not result in catch-up bone loss, at least for up to seven years after stopping treatment, but this may not be indefinite (Stevenson et al, 1992).

The view that the effects of HRT may wear off some time later is supported by other observations. In most communities hip fracture risk is greater in women than in men. The excess female risk increases progressively with age to a maximal value of twice that of the male risk at the age of 70 years (Elffors et al, 1994). Thereafter, the risk no longer increases. Similar observations have been made for other age-related fractures (Kanis and Pitt, 1992). The finite duration of the excess female morbidity for 20 years or so after the menopause, suggests a finite duration of the effect of

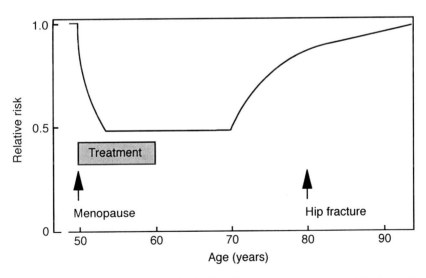

Figure 4. Relative risk of fracture associated with a 10-year treatment targeted at the time of the menopause. The treatment effect persists for 10 years after the withdrawal of treatment, and thereafter the effect progressively wears off so that by the median age of hip fracture (80 years), the efficacy has decreased from 50 to 10%. Reproduced from Kanis (1995, *American Journal of Medicine* **98** (supplement 2A):** 60–66) with permission.

the menopause. If true, this has important implication as it suggests that the impact of HRT is likely to be finite. Thus, 10 years of HRT at the menopause would have a progressively decreasing impact on hip and vertebral fractures after the age of 70 years, when most of the burden of osteoporosis falls in the elderly community (Johnell et al, 1993). Indeed, the attributable risk of menopause is low at the time of hip fracture (Johnell et al, 1995).

These considerations suggest that targetting HRT at the time of the menopause has less than optimal effects on osteoporotic fractures throughout the lifetime of women. Indeed, it may be preferable to target intervention specifically for osteoporosis at a time later in the natural history of the disorder. On the reasonable assumption that treatments are unlikely to be taken for life, and given that most hip fractures occur in the elderly, the effects of starting treatment later may have advantages. Similar benefits in terms of the number of hip fractures saved is achieved when treatment is instituted at the age of 70 years rather than at 50 years. If, however, a five-year treatment has a transient effect, irrespective of the age at which treatment is given, targetting intervention at the age of 70 years may actually save more hip fractures than targetting intervention at the time of the menopause (Johnell et al, 1993; Table 1). The use of HRT in the elderly should, therefore, be considered and the development of acceptable long-term HRT modalities in this age group will be an important area for research.

Table 1. Effect of different treatment strategies on the potential number of hip fractures saved. The model envisages increased use of oestrogens in a Swedish community from 15 to 25% of menopausal women. The risk of hip fracture is decreased by 50% for 10 years with a five-year treatment. Where a transient effect is modelled, efficacy wears off after stopping treatment (RR = 0.59 aged 60 to 64 years; RR = 0.67 aged 65 to 69 years and RR = 0.83 aged 70+ years). For additional assumptions see Johnell et al (1993).

Age (years)	Expected number of hip fractures	Number of fractures saved according to treatment			
		At menopause: Persistent effect	At menopause: Transient effect	At 70 years: Persistent effect	At 70 years: Transient effect
50–54	172	14	14	–	–
55–59	161	19	19	–	–
60–64	412	48	39	–	–
65–69	753	88	58	–	–
70–74	1348	157	52	157	157
75–79	2406	280	100	280	248
80–84	3116	362	130	362	260
85–89	2796	352	117	325	117
90+	1515	177	63	176	63
Total	12679	1470	592	1300	843
per cent of all fractures	100	11.6	4.6	10.2	6.6

IMPORTANCE OF GONADAL INSUFFICIENCY

The view that the vast majority of the problems of osteoporosis in women is due to the menopause ignores the importance of extragonadal factors; these factors are important in both men and women. A good example is the secular increase in all osteoporosis fractures that has occurred in many countries. These increases in age-specific risks with time affect men at least as much as women (Melton et al, 1987) and are clearly not dependent on oestrogen status. Further evidence for important extragonadal factors comes from epidemiological studies on hip fracture around the world. There are large inter-regional differences in the risk of fracture. In the case of hip fracture, this has been particularly well characterized from register and prospective multinational studies (Elffors et al, 1994). It is of interest that where the risk is high in women, so it is in men (Figure 5; Johnell et al, 1992). Indeed, there are greater differences in incidence between communities than there are differences between sexes within communities. This suggests that factors other than gonadal status are quantitatively more important in determining the heterogeneity of risk between communities. Moreover, there is a direct correlation between the age at menopause and the risk of hip fracture in ecological studies. Thus, the later the average age of menopause in a community, the higher the risk of hip fracture (Figure 6; Elffors et al, 1994). This should not be interpreted to suggest that a late menopause causes hip fracture (indeed the converse is true), but only that differences in menopausal age cannot account for the large differences in risk between communities.

These considerations suggest that the importance of the menopause to osteoporotic hip fracture risk has been overemphasized and that other factors are quantitatively more important in accounting for the regional differences in risk and the secular increases within many regions. These factors affect men as well as women and it will be important to identify these if substantial decreases in the burden of osteoporosis are to be achieved.

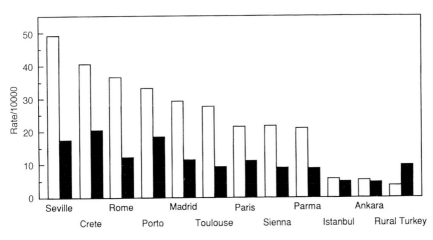

Figure 5. Age standardized risk for hip fracture in different European countries by sex. □, women; ■, men. Reproduced from Johnell et al (1992, *Osteoporosis International* **2**: 298–302) with permission.

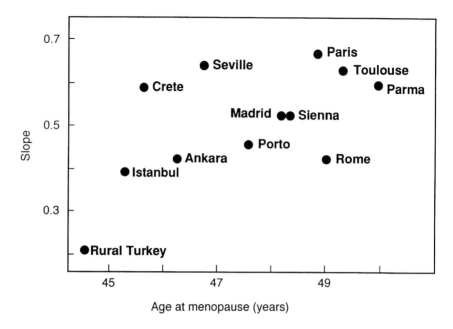

Figure 6. The risk of hip fracture in different countries (described as the increase in hip fracture risk with age, or slope) as a function of mean menopausal age. Hip fracture risk is higher in those communities with the menopause at a later age. Reproduced from Elffors et al (1994, *Osteoporosis International* **4**: 253–263) with permission.

SUMMARY

There is a persuasive rationale for the use of HRT at the time of the menopause, but there are a number of factors which limit its widespread application for osteoporosis. These relate partly to the long-term efficacy of HRT when given for a finite duration at the time of the menopause, and long-term prospective studies are warranted to address this issue. A further difficulty relates to the logic of targetting women at risk of osteoporosis at the time of the menopause when the benefits and risks of HRT are largely extraskeletal.

Finally, the importance of the menopause to the problems of osteoporosis have probably been overemphasized and other factors are important in determining the geographical variation in hip fracture risk as well as the increase in age- and sex-specific incidence that has occurred in many countries. The causes for this are unknown, but are clearly not related to gonadal status since these phenomena are observed both in men and in women. A plausible hypothesis is the decrease in physical activity, but this remains an hypothesis. It will be important to determine the aetiology of these phenomena so that logical preventive strategies can be developed.

REFERENCES

Anonymous (1993) Consensus Development Conference: Diagnosis, prophylaxis and treatment of osteoporosis. *American Journal of Medicine* **94:** 646–650.

Christiansen C, Nilas L, Riis B et al (1985) Uncoupling of bone formation and resorption by combined oestrogen and progestogen therapy in postmenopausal osteoporosis. *Lancet* **2.** 800–801.

Elffors L, Allander E, Kanis JA et al (1994) The variable incidence of hip fractures in Southern Europe. The MEDOS Study. *Osteoporosis International* **4:** 253–263.

Eriksen EF (1986) Normal and pathological remodelling of human trabecular bone: three dimensional reconstruction of the remodelling sequence in normals and in metabolic bone disease. *Endocrine Review* **7:** 379–408.

Garnett T, Savvas M & Studd JWW (1990) Reversal of bone loss with percutaneous oestrogens. In Drife JO & Studd JWW (Eds) *HRT and osteoporosis.* pp 295–314. London: Springer Verlag.

Grey A, Cundy T, Evans M & Reid I (1996) Medroxyprogesterone acetate enhances the spinal bone mineral density response to oestrogen in late postmenopausal women. *Clinical Endocrinology* (in press).

Johnell O, Gullberg B, Allander A & Kanis JA (1992) The apparent incidence of hip fracture in Europe: a study of national register sources. *Osteoporosis International* **2:** 298–302.

Johnell O, Stenbeck M, Rosen M et al (1993) Therapeutic strategies in the prevention of hip fractures with drugs affecting bone metabolism. *Bone* **14 (supplement 1):** S85–S87.

Johnell O, Gullberg B, Kanis JA et al (1995) Risk factors for hip fracture in European women: The MEDOS Study. *Journal of Bone Mineral Research* **10:** 1802–1815.

Kanis, JA (1984) Treatment of osteoporotic fracture. *Lancet* **i:** 27–33.

Kanis, JA (1991) The restoration of skeletal mass: A theoretic overview. *American Journal of Medicine* **91(5B):** 29–36.

Kanis JA (1995) Treatment of osteoporosis in elderly women. *American Journal of Medicine* **98 (supplement 2A):** 60–66.

Kanis JA & Pitt FA (1992) Epidemiology of osteoporosis. *Bone* **13 (supplement):** S7–S15.

Kanis JA & Stevenson JC (1994) Apparent offset of action of estrogens. *New England Journal of Medicine* **330:** 715.

Kanis JA, Melton LJ, Christiansen C et al (1994) The diagnosis of osteoporosis. *Journal of Bone Mineral Research* **9:** 1137–1141.

Law MR, Wald NJ & Meade TW (1991) Strategies for prevention of osteoporosis and hip fracture. *British Medical Journal* **303:** 453–459.

Lindsay R (1990) The pharmacology of estrogens. *Progress in Basic and Clinical Pharmacology* **4:** 55–72.

Lindsay R, Hart DM & Clark DM (1984) The minimum effective dose of oestrogen for prevention of postmenopausal bone loss. *Obstetrics and Gynecology* **63:** 754–763.

Lufkin EG, Wahner HW, O'Fallon WM et al (1992) Treatment of postmenopausal osteoporosis with transdermal estrogen. *Annals of Internal Medicine* **117:** 1–9.

Melton LJ, O'Fallon WM & Riggs BL (1987) Secular trends in the incidence of hip fractures. *Calcified Tissue International* **41:** 57–64.

Parfitt AM (1984) Age-related structural changes in trabecular and cortical bone: Cellular mechanisms and biomechanical consequences. *Calcified Tissue International* **36:** 122–128.

Stevenson JC, Kanis JA & Christiansen C (1992) Bone density measurement. *Lancet* **339:** 370–371.

World Health Organization (1994) Assessment of fracture risk and its application to screening for postmenopausal osteoporosis. *WHO Technical Report Series 843.* Geneva: WHO.

9

The menopause and the cardiovascular system

CAROLYN M. BEALE
PETER COLLINS

Cardiovascular disease (CVD) is often thought of as a disease associated with men rather than women, although epidemiological data do not support this view. Not only is death from CVD greater in women than men, but for women it is currently the most common cause of death. In the USA, CVD is responsible for the deaths of more women than cancer, accidents and diabetes combined (Eaker et al, 1993). However, whilst there is no basis for thinking that CVD is a disease restricted to men, there are clearly differences between the two sexes, especially with regard to age. In men, the incidence of CVD increases progressively from about the age of 35, whilst in women a rapid increase is not observed until after the age of 55 (Table 1). In the UK, for example in the age range from 35 to 39 years, mortality from coronary heart disease (CHD) is approximately sixfold lower in women than in men.

Table 1. Death rates from coronary heart disease in women in England and Wales in 1993 by age group.

Age group	Deaths per 1000 women
45–54	1.2
55–64	4.6
65–74	12.4

Source = Office of Population Censuses and Surveys, series DH2 number 20.

CARDIOVASCULAR DISEASE IN WOMEN

Risk and the menopause

Since the original observation that CVD rarely affects women before the menopause, oestrogen deficiency has been strongly implicated in the aetiology of the disease.

Analysis of data from a large prospective cohort study of 121 700 women strongly supports the role of oestrogen in reducing the risk for CVD (Colditz et al, 1987). After adjusting for age and cigarette smoking, women

Baillière's Clinical Obstetrics and Gynaecology—
Vol. 10, No. 3, September 1996
ISBN 0–7020–2177–6
0950–3552/96/030483 + 32 $12.00/00

who had undergone bilateral oophorectomy and who had not taken oestrogen after the menopause were found to have a significantly increased risk of CHD (relative risk 2.2), whilst the post-menopausal use of oestrogen replacement therapy (ORT) appeared to counter this effect and reduced the risk to 0.9 (Figure 1).

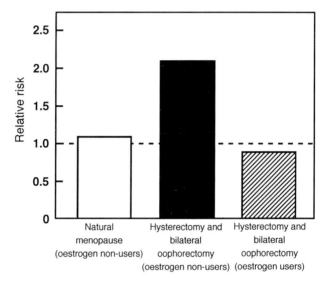

Figure 1. The increased risk from baseline for coronary heart disease for women who had undergone bilateral oophorectomy was sixfold that of women experiencing a natural menopause. Oestrogen replacement significantly reduced the relative risk. Adapted from Colditz et al (1987).

Risk factors for heart disease in women

The risk factors for heart disease in women and men are similar (Table 2), however psychosocial and menopausal factors play an important role in women.

Table 2. Relative contribution of risk for heart disease in women.

Risk factor	Odds ratio
Smoking	4.9
Diabetes	4.5
Cholesterol > 240 mg/l	2.1
Family history	1.9
Hypertension	1.3
Obesity	1.1
Oestrogen therapy	0.5

Psychosocial stress

Stress in pre-menopausal women can interfere with the ovarian cycle which may represent a risk factor for CVD. Studies in cynomolgus monkeys that were chronically stressed showed that coronary artery atherosclerosis was indistinguishable from male monkeys and post-menopausal female monkeys (Shively and Clarkson, 1994). In these monkeys the mechanism for atherosclerotic development is linked to ovarian dysfunction leading to oestrogen deprivation (Clarkson, 1994). Chronic stress in monkeys causes them to have normal menstrual cycles but the peak oestradiol levels are about a quarter of those of normal levels (Williams et al, 1994). Stress could therefore theoretically adversely affect coronary heart disease risk in women.

Cigarette smoking

Cigarette smoking may be more deleterious in women than men. Smoking results in an earlier menopause, a decrease in high density lipoprotein cholesterol (HDL-C) with an increase in platelet aggregability and fibrinogen levels. Cessation of smoking results in a reduction in risk of cardiac events within three to four years, almost nearly to that of a non-smoker (Rosenberg et al, 1990).

Diabetes

A diabetic woman is at high risk of developing CVD (Abbott et al, 1987), and this is a more important risk for women than for men (Brezinka and Padmos, 1994; Rich-Edwards et al, 1995). Diabetes appears to eliminate the cardio-protective effects of oestrogen and the increase in risk of CVD for a woman with diabetes is three to four times that of a healthy woman. Diabetics have a greater post-myocardial infarction and intervention morbidity and mortality.

Blood pressure

No reliable prospective, randomized study exists which investigates the effect of hormone replacement therapy (HRT) on blood pressure. An observational study of oestrogen use and stroke risk in post-menopausal women demonstrated a significant association between oestrogen use and hypertension (Pfeffer and van den Noort, 1976). However, subsequent studies have observed no difference in blood pressure between post-menopausal oestrogen users and non-users over a five-month period (Pfeffer et al, 1979) and a five-year follow-up period (Hammond et al, 1979). The Postmenopausal Estrogen/Progestin Interventions (PEPI) study supports these findings because systolic blood pressure in the treated groups was not significantly different from the placebo group (Anonymous, 1995).

The risk of the development of hypertension with ORT whether un-opposed or given with added progestogen, is low. The few cases of oestrogen-induced hypertension which have been reported are thought to represent rare idiosyncratic reactions to oestrogen.

Hypertension

The cardiovascular effects of hypertension may be reduced in female patients, but there is still a strong association between hypertension and cardiovascular morbidity and mortality in women (Brezinka and Padmos, 1994; Rich-Edwards et al, 1995). The development of left ventricular hypertrophy and diastolic dysfunction is an important indicator of increased risk. The presence of left ventricular hypertrophy is an important variable in predicting long-term prognosis in patients with hypertension.

Hazzard (1989) noted that the most carefully designed studies suggested that blood pressure was consistently, although minimally, lowered by oestrogen administration (Lind et al, 1979; Luotola, 1983). One study (Lip et al, 1994) found no effect of HRT on blood pressure in patients with hypertension. Therefore, the assumption that HRT aggravates hypertension is not substantiated by the evidence to date, however there still remains a need for randomized studies in this area.

It is therefore inappropriate to caution the use of HRT in patients with hypertension, although idiosyncratic reactions may rarely occur.

CHD in women

Information on CHD shows that not only do women present with the disease later in life than men, but they more frequently present with angina and less frequently with sudden death. CVDs are also a major cause of disability in women. In 1980, the percentage of women with ischaemic heart disease who were disabled by the disease was 36% in women aged 55 to 64 and 55% in women aged 75 and older. For women surviving a stroke the situation is even worse, with over 60% of women over the age of 54 suffering some form of disability (Eaker et al, 1993). The fact that CVD is as much a problem for women as for men is not, however, reflected in treatment patterns. Although women experience chest pain as the main symptom of coronary artery disease more frequently than men, fewer women are referred for non-invasive tests. Studies, both in Europe and North America, have shown that men with significant CHD are more likely than women to undergo revascularization. Although there are a number of logical factors that might explain this apparent difference, there is some evidence that despite the greater incidence of disability associated with CVD in women, physicians tend to pursue a less aggressive approach to the management and treatment of coronary disease in women as compared to men (Steingart et al, 1991).

Diagnosing chest pain in women

Angina in women is more difficult to evaluate than in men. Younger women have a lower prevalence of CHD and there is a greater chance of tests, such as the exercise test, being abnormal in the absence of significant obstructive CHD. The reliance on tests such as the exercise test can be deceptive, since the specificity and sensitivity are reduced in females. In older women with a classical history of exertional angina pectoris and associated risk factors, the specificity and the exercise test sensitivity is increased.

Presentation of CHD in women

Because of the later development of CHD in women, men tend to present at a younger age than women. Most women initially present in their 70s or 80s (Table 1). In contrast to men, women present more frequently with angina pectoris and with myocardial infarction (65% versus 35%). Symptoms may be ignored by physicians, delaying investigation. Over 30% of women present with sudden cardiac death or fatal myocardial infarction. If the Rose questionnaire is used to assess angina (Rose and Blackburn, 1968)—defined as chest pain with characteristics suggesting that it arises from the heart—it is more common in women than in men. However, a history of classical, exercise related angina may turn out to be more common in men. The initial presentation in women is more urgent (since it is usually delayed) than in men who tend to be referred under elective conditions.

Myocardial infarction

Evidence suggests that women seek medical help later than men on presentation of myocardial infarction. The reason for this is not entirely clear (Clarke et al, 1994).

Oestrogen and the cardiological syndrome X in females

Angina pectoris is usually caused by obstructive atheromatous coronary artery disease. Angiographically smooth coronary arteries are found in approximately 20% of patients who undergo coronary angiography (Likoff et al, 1967; Phibbs et al, 1988). The majority of these patients are women (Turiel et al, 1987; Cannon and Epstein, 1988). The triad of angina pectoris, a positive exercise test, and angiographically smooth coronary arteries, is commonly referred to as syndrome X, a term first used by Kemp et al (1973). The pathophysiology of the troublesome chest pain in syndrome X is poorly understood, and there are many suggested mechanisms (Cannon and Epstein, 1988; Maseri et al, 1991; Rosano et al, 1991). Although syndrome X is likely to be a heterogeneous condition, reduced coronary flow reserve induced by dipyridamole has been reported in many patients with this diagnosis (Opherk et al, 1981; Cannon and Epstein, 1988). Most of the women with syndrome X are post-menopausal (Kaski et al, 1995). Indeed, oestrogen deficiency is associated with vasomotor instability and decreased arterial blood flow velocity in humans (Kronenberg et al, 1984; Rees and Barlow, 1988; Sullivan et al, 1988; Ginsburg and Hardiman, 1989).

A recent study has investigated the clinical and gynaecological features of female patients with syndrome X in order to ascertain whether ovarian hormone deficiency plays a role in unmasking the syndrome in female patients (Figure 2) (Rosano et al, 1995). Another study has shown that oestrogen may be helpful in the treatment of this condition (Rosano et al, 1996).

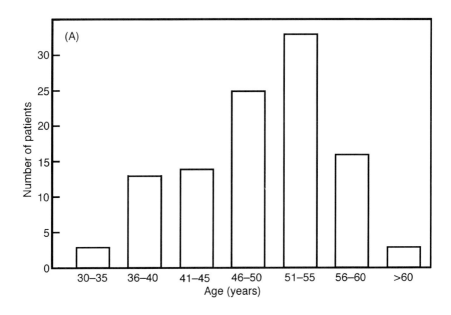

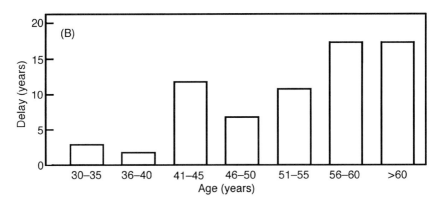

Figure 2. (A) Onset of chest pain, by age, in 107 women with syndrome X. Most of the women were either perimenopausal or menopausal. (B) Time delay to onset of chest pain following hysterectomy in 43 women with syndrome X. In younger women the delay was shorter implying that the syndrome may be precipitated by abrupt changes in plasma oestradiol levels.

Epidemiology of CHD in women

The fact that heart disease increases rapidly in women during the climacteric, and that women who have undergone bilateral oophorectomy have an increased risk of atherosclerosis and CHD is strongly suggestive that ORT can decrease the risk of developing and dying from heart disease. Considerable epidemiological evidence supports this hypothesis. In a review of population-based case-control studies, cross-sectional studies and prospective studies of ORT and CHD, Stampfer and Colditz (1991) calculated that the overall relative risk associated with ORT was reduced to 0.56. Only the Framingham study reported an elevated risk (Gordon et al, 1978); however re-analysis of this data revealed a non-significant protective effect in younger women and a non-significant increase in risk in older women (Stampfer and Colditz, 1991).

It is now clear, both from clinical research and from epidemiological studies, that ORT has the potential to significantly reduce the risk of CVD. The precise mode of action of this cardioprotective effect remains uncertain, but it is now known that many factors are involved, including favourable changes in cardiovascular risk factors as well as direct effects on the vascular system.

Evidence that post-menopausal HRT protects the cardiovascular system

There are a number of published reports of large epidemiological studies which include many women over long periods of time. There are over 30 studies reporting on the effect of HRT on the risk of CVD, using recognizable endpoints. Owing to the early and widespread use of conjugated oestrogens, especially in the USA, most of the oestrogen exposure relates to conjugated oestrogens. The studies are from different sources and different countries, mainly the USA, the UK and Scandinavia and are largely consistent. Further evidence is derived from studies on risk factors for CVD.

A number of endpoints have been investigated in observational trials with HRT.

Myocardial infarction

Studies which investigated the effect of ORT on the risk of myocardial infarction demonstrated a reduced risk from ORT (Rosenberg et al, 1976; Jick et al, 1978; Pfeffer et al, 1978; Nachtigall et al, 1979; Adam et al, 1981; Bain et al, 1981; Szklo et al, 1984; Lafferty and Helmuth, 1985; Stampfer et al, 1985; Henderson et al, 1986, 1988, 1991; Petitti et al, 1987; Croft and Hannaford, 1989a; Falkeborn et al, 1992; Lafferty and Fiske, 1994; Psaty et al, 1994). The studies which included combination therapy with oestrogens and progestogens also indicated a protective effect (Falkeborn et al, 1992; Lafferty and Fiske, 1994; Psaty et al, 1994).

Stroke

A majority of the studies reporting on the effect of ORT on the risk of stroke showed a reduction in risk (Byrd et al, 1977; Adam et al, 1981; Stampfer et al, 1985; Wilson et al, 1985; Bush et al, 1987; Petitti et al, 1987; Paganini-Hill et al, 1988; Hunt et al, 1990; Henderson et al, 1991; Falkeborn et al, 1993). A smaller number showed no change (Pfeffer and van den Noort, 1976; Rosenberg et al, 1980; Lafferty and Fiske, 1994) and one (Wilson et al, 1985) showed an increase in risk. Three studies (Paganini-Hill et al, 1988; Henderson et al, 1991; Finucane et al, 1993) which estimated death from stroke, showed a significant reduction in risk. Grady et al (1992) pooled 15 studies and estimated that the relative risk for stroke from all studies was 0.96 (95% CI 0.82–1.13). Two studies (Falkeborn et al, 1993; Lafferty and Fiske, 1994) reported on the effects of oestrogen in combination with progestogen. Both studies showed no increase in the risk of stroke.

All cause mortality and CVD

A number of studies (Burch et al, 1974; Byrd et al, 1977; Wilson et al, 1985; Bush et al, 1987; Petitti et al, 1987; Criqui et al, 1988; Hunt et al, 1990; Henderson et al, 1991; Stampfer et al, 1991) investigated the effect of ORT on all-cause mortality. All except one (Wilson et al, 1985) were consistent in demonstrating reduced mortality in oestrogen users. Studies (Burch et al, 1974; Byrd et al, 1977; Ross et al, 1981; Stampfer et al, 1985; Bush et al, 1987; Petitti et al, 1987; Criqui et al, 1988; Paganini-Hill et al, 1988; Hunt et al, 1990; Henderson et al, 1991) which investigated the effect on mortality from CVD demonstrated a reduction in risk.

Reduction of coronary atherosclerosis

Three studies (Gruchow et al, 1988; Sullivan et al, 1988; McFarland et al, 1989) have demonstrated that coronary occlusion as measured by coronary angiography, is reduced in women taking oestrogen at the time of cardiac catheterization. All studies were consistent in showing significant reduction in coronary artery disease in post-menopausal oestrogen users. Sullivan et al (1990) also reported that women with CHD who had had HRT had a significantly better prognosis following angiography.

Surgical menopause

A number of studies have demonstrated reduction in the risk of CVD in women with surgical menopause (Byrd et al, 1977; Bain et al, 1981; Szklo et al, 1984; Colditz et al, 1987; McFarland et al, 1989; Stampfer et al, 1991). Three studies (Bain et al, 1981; McFarland et al, 1989; Stampfer et al, 1991) showed greater protection in women with a surgical menopause compared with women with a natural menopause.

Cigarette smoking

ORT appears to decrease the risk of CVD in cigarette smokers (Ross et al, 1981; Wilson et al, 1985; Bush et al, 1987; Criqui et al, 1988; Henderson et al, 1988, 1991; Sullivan et al, 1988). Overall, the studies showed that conjugated oestrogens had no adverse interaction with cigarette smoking which increased the risk of CVD. All except one demonstrated a protective effect in post-menopausal cigarette smokers.

Reduction of risk in higher risk women

Separate analyses were made in four studies (Ross et al, 1981; Bush et al, 1987; Henderson et al, 1988, 1991) to estimate the effect of post-menopausal ORT in subjects who were at high risk of CVD because of a previous history of angina, myocardial infarction, stroke, diabetes, hypertension, or raised lipid levels. These studies showed that protection was conferred in the high risk groups which were studied.

Combined oestrogen and progestogen

An oestrogen-progestogen combination has also been shown to reduce the risk of CVD in post-menopausal women. Seven studies (Ross et al, 1981; Wilson et al, 1985; Bush et al, 1987; Criqui et al, 1988; Henderson et al, 1988, 1991; Sullivan et al, 1988) have demonstrated a reduction in the risk of CVD when progestogens were added to ORT.

Meta-analyses of the epidemiological data

Stampfer and Colditz (1991) reviewed 31 studies on the effect of ORT on CHD (Table 3) and concluded that the bulk of the evidence strongly suggested a protective effect that was unlikely to be explained by confounding factors. When all studies were combined in a meta-analysis the relative risk was calculated as 0.56 (95% CI 0.50–0.61). The estimated relative risks were weighted proportionally to the precision of the study. The larger studies with more precise estimates and narrower confidence limits were given greater weight than the smaller ones. An estimate of variance was derived when necessary by calculating the standard error from the confidence interval of each study. Barrett-Connor and Bush (1991)

Table 3. Results of a meta-analysis of observational studies on coronary heart disease and use of oestrogen replacement therapy, by category of study design. Source, Stampfer and Colditz (1991).

Study design	RR	CI (95%)
Hospital-based case-control studies	1.33	0.93–1.91
Population-based case-control studies	0.76	0.61–0.94
Cohort with external controls studies	0.36	0.28–0.47
Cohort with internal controls studies	0.58	0.48–0.69
Cross-sectional angiography studies	0.41	0.34–0.50

reviewed the evidence from 18 studies and weighted the risk estimate from each study for study type, study size and recency of oestrogen use. The estimate of the reduction in risk was 40–50%.

Grady's meta-analysis (Grady et al, 1992) based on 32 studies on the effect of ORT on CHD estimated a relative risk of 0.65 (95% CI 0.59–0.71).

Studies on risk factors for CVD

The PEPI study (Anonymous, 1995) compared different regimens of HRT with placebo in 875 post-menopausal women aged 45–64. The women were randomly assigned to five groups and treated with placebo, 0.625 mg conjugated oestrogens daily, 0.625 mg conjugated oestrogens daily plus 10 mg medroxyprogesterone acetate (MPA) for 12 days in each month, or 0.625 mg conjugated oestrogens plus 200 mg micronized progesterone for 12 days in each month. Oestrogen alone or with a progestogen improved lipoproteins and lowered fibrinogen levels without detectable effects on post-challenge insulin or blood pressure.

Manolio et al (1993) reported on a sample of 2,955 women aged 65–100 who were included in a cardiovascular health study in four USA communities. Among the 2,955 women interviewed, 356 (12%) were currently using oestrogen or combined oestrogen and progestogen. A total of 281 (79%) were taking unopposed oestrogen. An additional 784 (26.5%) women reported past use of hormones. The median duration of use was 18 years in current users and three years in past users. Past or present use of oestrogen was strongly associated with favourable risk factor profiles. Oestrogen users had higher HDL-C and factor VII, and lower low density lipoprotein cholesterol (LDL-C), fibrinogen, fasting insulin and glucose. Similar associations of oestrogen use with risk factors were seen in younger and older women and smokers and non-smokers.

The more recent MRC study (MRC Working Party, 1992) is a randomized double-blind study including 321 hysterectomized women aged 35–59. Women were assigned to two groups and treated with 0.625 mg conjugated oestrogens daily or 0.625 mg conjugated oestrogens daily plus 150 µg norgestrel for 12 days in each month. The women treated with unopposed conjugated oestrogens or conjugated oestrogens with norgestrel had decreased total cholesterol and LDL-C levels. HDL-C levels rose to significantly higher levels in women taking oestrogen alone, but triglycerides and factor VII activity were also higher in this group. Fibrinogen was decreased in both treated groups. From these data, the authors suggested that oestrogen/progestogen therapy may be as cardio-protective as oestrogen given alone, and there appear to be no adverse effects on metabolic parameters. Combined therapy may be the regimen of choice in hysterectomized as well as unhysterectomized women.

What does the epidemiological evidence mean?

There is a large and consistent body of evidence from the cited observational studies showing a positive beneficial association between the use of HRT and reduced risk of CHD. The numbers of women reported in these studies would strongly support that these results are not due to chance. The large cohort studies report a relative risk reduction of 50%; this would translate to an absolute reduction in CHD mortality of about six women per 1,000 per year aged 65–74. In support of the epidemiological studies, results from metabolic and risk factor studies show favourable lipid, metabolic and haemostatic profiles relating to HRT.

The case that HRT is cardioprotective rests on the results of observational studies and not randomized trials. It has been suggested that these studies are flawed because they may contain biases such as selection bias and confounding. There is almost a universal opinion which criticizes observational studies in this way, the belief being that randomized controlled trials are the only valid form of evidence of efficacy. The alternative however, is to critically review evidence from observational studies, especially when the results of trials will not be available for over a decade (as is the case for HRT).

Selection bias will occur when subjects studied are not representative of patients with a particular characteristic in the target population. Controls for the larger studies however are drawn from the same cohort (Bush et al, 1987; Stampfer et al, 1991), thus nullifying any effect of selection.

Confounding has been suggested as a reason for the favourable effect of HRT; that is, women who take hormones genuinely have fewer CHD events than other women. Some variables in unselected populations do exist such as users being from a higher social class, exercise more, are less overweight and visit health professionals more. These reported differences are usually small in degree and are often statistically insignificant (Hemminki and Sihvo, 1993). To counter this claim, some extremely important variables, such as cigarette smoking, do not appear to be different between users and non-users.

Explaining away the apparent risk reduction due to HRT as the result of confounding is biologically inconsistent. Women taking HRT in the observational cohort studies had different lipid profiles from non-users. These differences have been reproduced in randomized controlled trials. If the lipid changes induced by HRT were a true effect it is not entirely plausible to claim that differences in CHD outcome are purely due to confounding.

The existence of smaller differences in risk due to residual confounding is impossible to exclude. There may therefore be an over estimation of the size of the true benefit of taking HRT. Sufficient evidence has accumulated showing that HRT does protect against CVD in women, although data regarding the true magnitude of that protection remain incomplete (Lip et al, 1995).

POSSIBLE MECHANISMS OF ACTION OF HRT REDUCING CARDIOVASCULAR RISK

The loss of ovarian function at the menopause and the resulting decrease in plasma oestrogen levels has significant detrimental effects on risk factors for CVD. Therefore, ORT may reverse the negative effect of the menopause on cardiovascular risk.

Metabolic risk factors

Lipids

Large scale studies attribute 30–50% of the cardioprotective effect of oestrogen to a beneficial effect on lipid profile (Stampfer and Colditz, 1991). Women aged 20 to 50 years have a more favourable lipid profile than men of a similar age (lower plasma LDL-C and very low-density lipoprotein (VLDL), and higher plasma HDL-C). However, at the menopause there is an associated detrimental change in lipid profile, namely an increase in LDL-C and a concurrent decrease in HDL-C (Stevenson et al, 1993). This change is reversed with ORT, with the HDL_2 subclass of the HDL-C fraction being particularly beneficially affected. HDL_2 is most strongly associated with coronary atherosclerosis (a negative association) (Godsland et al, 1987).

Lipoprotein(a) (Lp(a)) has been suggested as an important risk factor for coronary artery disease, with high levels being associated with increased risk, as it plays an important role in reverse cholesterol transport (removal of cholesterol from the systemic circulation) (Godsland et al, 1987). ORT in post-menopausal women lowers plasma Lp(a), as does combined oestrogen/progestogen therapy (Nabulsi et al, 1993; Soma et al, 1991), and in this way may exert a partial beneficial effect on cardiovascular risk.

There has been concern over reports that ORT may cause a potentially detrimental elevation of plasma triglyceride levels (Barrett-Connor et al,

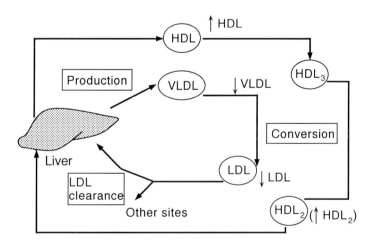

Figure 3. Oestrogen replacement therapy reverses the adverse changes in lipid metabolism associated with the menopause by increasing the levels of high density lipoproteins (HDL) and their subfractions and decreasing the levels of low density lipoproteins (LDL).

1989; Lobo, 1991; Walsh et al, 1991; Nabulsi et al, 1993). However the cardiovascular relevance of this increase is questionable. Oestrogen appears to enhance the synthesis of VLDL triglycerides in the liver, particularly large, triglyceride rich VLDL (Walsh et al, 1991). Large VLDL is catabolized by the liver and is not converted to VLDL and LDL-C, therefore having a less sinister effect on cardiovascular risk than other triglycerides. The addition of a progestogen to ORT has little or no effect on triglyceride levels (Figure 3) (Nabulsi et al, 1993).

In summary, ORT has a beneficial effect on lipid profile by lowering LDL-C and increasing plasma HDL-C, with no apparent significant effect on plasma triglyceride levels. The addition of a progestogen to ORT does little to negate the beneficial effect of ORT and, indeed, combined therapy may be more beneficial to cardiovascular risk than ORT alone (Nabulsi et al, 1993).

Insulin resistance

It is well known that diabetes is strongly associated with CHD, and diabetic women have a higher incidence of this than diabetic men (Abbott et al, 1987). Insulin resistance can be defined as a relative decrease in the sensitivity of target tissue to the action of insulin with an associated increase in circulating insulin concentrations. Hyperinsulinaemia resulting from insulin resistance is associated with increased cardiovascular risk. Glucose metabolism deteriorates with increasing age (Stevenson et al, 1994), and is also affected by the menopause, although there may be difficulties in discerning change due to the menopause from change attributed to age.

HRT has a beneficial effect on insulin resistance. Oral conjugated equine oestrogens do not significantly affect carbohydrate metabolism (Cagnacci et al, 1992). Oral preparations result in high steroid concentrations in the liver (Godsland et al, 1993). Because the liver is also a major site of insulin processing and action it is possible that the transdermal route is more favourable than the oral route in insulin and glucose metabolism because of a lesser impact on the liver.

There is no evidence of an increased incidence of diabetes in association with HRT. Some metabolic studies indicated some favourable and some unfavourable changes. The changes were small and their importance is unknown.

Haemostasis

Thrombogenesis plays an important role in the pathogenesis and presentation of CHD, and haemostatic factors are an important factor in this. The menopause has a variety of effects on haemostasis. The procoagulant factor VII levels increase (Scarabin et al, 1990), as do plasma fibrinogen (Folsom et al, 1991) and tissue plasminogen activator levels, indicating an increased risk of arterial thrombosis due to hypercoagulability. Plasminogen activator inhibitor-1 (PAI-1), a factor which is negatively related to fibrinolysis, is also elevated in post-menopausal women (Heinrich et al, 1991). Studies confirm that oestrogen status is associated with increased fibrinolytic potential (Gebara et al, 1995). However, there is no evidence to suggest any overall change in fibrin generation or degradation, and no increase in thrombin generation which may be attributed to the menopause (Pinto et al, 1990).

Limited epidemiological studies and extensive studies on the effects of oestrogen on the haemostatic system in post-menopausal women indicate no evidence of adverse effects on coagulation parameters. There are no data to support the fact that post-menopausal ORT increases the risk of venous thromboembolism. The reduction in fibrinogen is favourable. The evidence does not suggest an adverse effect of HRT, with oestrogens alone or combined with progestogens, on the coagulation cascade.

DIRECT VASCULAR EFFECTS OF OESTROGEN ON THE VASCULAR SYSTEM

Sex hormones are vasoactive substances which affect the vasculature of many systems as well as the reproductive vascular system. Oestrogen relaxes animal and human coronary and cerebral arteries and it could be that the cardioprotective role of HRT is partially mediated through direct effects on the vascular system, although the mechanism(s) involved are still to be fully elucidated.

Vascular resistance and blood flow

In the oestrogen-deplete state, local and systemic administration of 17β-oestradiol has effects on both reproductive and non-reproductive vascular beds (Magness and Rosenfeld, 1989). The effect of acute and chronic oestrogen administration on systemic haemodynamics has been studied in post-menopausal women. Acute administration of sublingual 17β-oestradiol affects the peripheral vasculature in humans. Forty minutes after the administration of sublingual 17β-oestradiol to post-menopausal volunteers there was an increase in forearm blood flow and a reduction in forearm vascular resistance compared to placebo, with no difference in mean arterial blood pressure (Volterrani et al, 1995). Forearm vasodilatation induced by acetylcholine can also be potentiated by the acute local administration of intravenous oestradiol in healthy post-menopausal women (Gilligan et al, 1994a). Aortic peak flow velocity gradually decreases with time since the onset of the menopause (Pines et al, 1992), and there is a significant increase in aortic flow velocity and acceleration after 10 weeks of HRT (Pines et al, 1991). Long-term treatment with 17β-oestradiol (22 weeks) in normotensive post-menopausal women results in a decrease in pulsatility index of the carotid artery, thought to represent impedance to blood flow (Ganger et al, 1991). Physiological doses of oestrogen were used in this study and the resulting effect took several weeks to become apparent. The fall in pulsatility index with oestrogen treatment correlated with the duration since the menopause. These peripheral vascular effects may involve one or a number of mechanisms of action of oestrogen. The mechanisms may differ depending on the dose of oestrogen used and the duration of use and whether used in combination with a progestogen (Ganger et al, 1991; Volterrani et al, 1995).

Vascular function—potential mechanisms

A number of mechanisms have been proposed to explain the direct vascular effects of oestrogen. The present evidence suggests that the mechanisms responsible for acute vascular and chronic cardioprotective effects may differ. Oestrogen has direct effects on the smooth muscle of blood vessels resulting in direct vascular relaxation. There are also indirect relaxing effects of oestrogen via the endothelium, by stimulation of nitric oxide synthase, resulting in an increased synthesis and release of nitric oxide (NO).

Recent human studies have investigated the acute direct effects of oestrogen on the coronary arteries, implicating a role of the endothelium in oestrogen-induced coronary relaxation (Collins et al, 1994, 1995; Gilligan et al, 1994b; Reis et al, 1994; Chester et al, 1995). However, with long-term therapy other mechanisms may be involved—calcium antagonism and inhibition of atherogenesis have been suggested (Jiang et al, 1992a; Collins et al, 1993). Oestrogen has also been shown to affect prostaglandin production and affect constrictor factors like endothelin (Magness et al, 1992; Muck et al, 1993; Polderman et al, 1993). Some of the acute vascular effects of oestrogen may be independent of the classical oestrogen receptor, although receptor-dependence may be involved in long-term vascular protection. Further research is necessary to demonstrate the relevance of these various mechanisms in the long-term cardioprotective effect of HRT in post-menopausal women, with and without pre-existing CVD.

Direct effects of oestrogen on the coronary arteries

17β-Oestradiol has direct smooth muscle, endothelium-independent, relaxing effects on coronary blood vessels. In isolated rabbit coronary arteries Jiang et al (1991) demonstrated direct vascular smooth muscle relaxation with 17β-oestradiol. Important differences in the relaxation response of isolated human coronary arteries to oestrogen have recently been published (Figure 4) (Mügge et al, 1993; Chester et al, 1995). Relaxation was significantly greater in coronary arteries from female compared to male patients. No significant differences were seen between arteries with or without endothelium nor after nitric oxide synthase (NOS) or cyclooxygenase inhibition. These results indicate that 17β-oestradiol induces human coronary artery relaxation by an endothelium-independent mechanism in vitro. The gender of the patients significantly affects sensitivity of the coronary arterial rings to oestrogen. The mechanism(s) or importance of this finding remains to be determined.

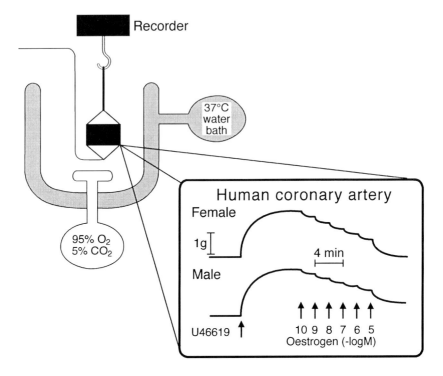

Figure 4. Precontracted human coronary arteries in vitro can be relaxed by oestradiol. Coronary arteries from females are more sensitive than those from males.

Mechanisms of vascular smooth muscle relaxation

Calcium antagonism

Pharmacological evidence for a calcium antagonistic mechanism has been identified in isolated rabbit coronary arteries (Jiang et al, 1991). More recently this has been confirmed in coronary vascular myocytes (Jiang et al, 1992a) and isolated smooth muscle myocytes (Han et al, 1995) by measuring contraction, cytosolic calcium concentration and calcium currents (Jiang et al, 1991, 1992a; Han et al, 1995).

It has been hypothesized that some of the cardiovascular benefits of ORT may be due to a calcium antagonist effect of oestrogen (Collins et al, 1993). In a long-term study of oestrogen in atherosclerotic, ovariectomized cynomolgus monkeys, a decrease in coronary atheroma was reported compared to the non-treated animals (Adams et al, 1990). Long-term calcium antagonist treatment is known to decrease the progression of atheroma when given to patients with established CHD (Lichtlen et al, 1990; Waters et al, 1990), therefore oestrogen may have a beneficial effect on atheroma progression due to its calcium antagonistic properties in vivo.

Endothelium-dependent and NO-dependent relaxation

The endothelium, a monolayer of cells which lines the intimal surface of the entire circulatory system, plays an important role in the modulation of coronary tone by formation and secretion of a large number of substances. Endothelium-derived relaxing factor (EDRF), now known to be NO or a closely related substance (Palmer et al, 1987; Myers et al, 1989), is one of these substances.

NO causes vasorelaxation in endothelium-intact coronary arteries and is a product of the conversion of L-arginine by NOS to NO and citrulline. NOS can be divided into two functional groups based on calcium sensitivity. Oestrogen can induce calcium-dependent NOS, thus enhancing the amount of available NOS in a cell (Weiner et al, 1994). NO has also been observed to slow the development of atheroma by inhibiting smooth muscle cell proliferation while stimulating proliferation of endothelial cells (Dubey and Overbeck, 1994). Oestrogen is a potent antioxidant of lipids (Sack et al, 1994), and oxidized lipids inhibit NO (Simon et al, 1990). Oestrogen may therefore be cardioprotective via enhanced NO production or reversal of its inhibition which in turn has antiatherogenic properties. The time course for this effect is unknown and may be relevant only with long-term oestrogen treatment. An increased basal release of NO in endothelium-intact aortic rings from female rabbits than those from males has been reported (Hayashi et al, 1992), and oestrogen-induced increases in blood flow in the uterine artery can be antagonized by NOS inhibition (Van Buren et al, 1992). Oestrogen can stimulate constitutive NOS in cultured bovine endothelial cells (Schray-Utz et al, 1993). Experiments in cultured monolayers of human umbilical vein demonstrate that oestrogen stimulates basal NOS sixfold within 30 minutes (Figure 5) (Caulin-Glaser et al, 1994).

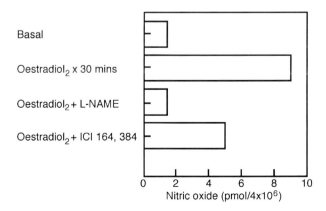

Figure 5. Cultured monolayers of human umbilical vein demonstrated that nitric oxide production can be stimulated sixfold by oestradiol within 30 minutes. Adapted from Caulin-Glaser et al (1994).

This stimulation was inhibited by specific oestrogen receptor antagonism. An acute effect on the constitutive enzyme is possible and may account for some of the acute blood flow responses to oestrogen in vivo. An in vivo study in guinea pigs examined the effects of oestrogen on NOS activity in heart, kidney and skeletal muscle. Oestradiol increased NO in female guinea pigs after five days' treatment, however this occurred in males only after 10 days of oestrogen exposure (Figure 6) (Weiner et al, 1994). This

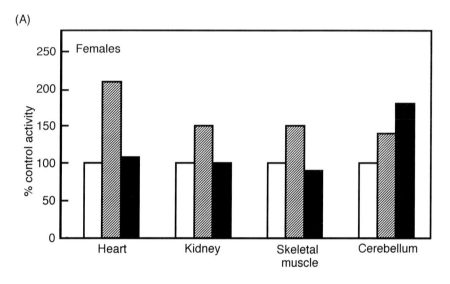

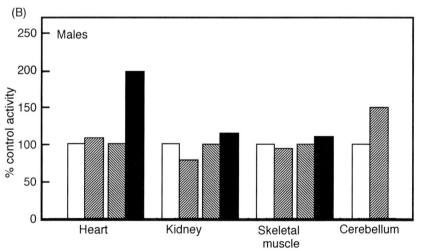

Figure 6. Calcium-dependent nitric oxide synthase stimulation by the sex hormones in (A) females (□, control; ▨, oestradiol₂; ■, testosterone) and (B) males (5-day: □, control; ▨, oestradiol₂; 10-day: ▨, control; ■, oestradiol₂). Adapted from Weiner et al (1994).

effect was inhibited by tamoxifen. These two studies suggest that the classical oestrogen receptor is involved in the stimulation of NOS. It was suggested that the number or availability of oestrogen receptors in male tissues is initially too low requiring a period of oestrogen priming.

Possible in vivo endothelium-dependent effects of oestrogen

Oestrogen-induced, NO-dependent, increases in uterine blood flow in animals in vivo can be inhibited by L-NAME, an antagonist of NO production (Van Buren et al, 1992). This confirms in some vascular beds in vivo that oestrogen-induced endothelium-dependent increases in blood flow can occur.

Studies in oestrogen-deficient female monkeys show that atherosclerosis impairs acetylcholine-mediated vascular responses (Williams et al, 1990, 1992). Two-year treatment with oestrogen protects against impaired vascular responses of atherosclerotic coronary arteries to acetylcholine in post-menopausal female monkeys (Williams et al, 1990). In an acute study, coronary angiography in monkeys with coronary atherosclerosis demonstrated that arteries constricted in response to intracoronary infusion of acetylcholine before oestrogen treatment, but dilated 20 minutes after intravenous infusion of ethinyl oestradiol (Williams et al, 1992).

In humans, the endothelium may be involved in the mediation of oestrogen-induced coronary relaxation. Although oestrogen has little effect directly, it does attenuate (Reis et al, 1994), or abolish (Gilligan et al, 1994b; Collins et al, 1995), acetylcholine-induced vasoconstriction when administered acutely (15 to 20 minutes after bolus or continuous intracoronary infusion) in post-menopausal women with atherosclerotic coronary arteries. An increase in coronary blood flow and cross-sectional area, and decreased resistance in post-menopausal women occurred 15 minutes after an intravenous infusion of ethinyl oestradiol. Abnormal coronary vasomotor responses to acetylcholine were attenuated. Similar reversal of acetylcholine-induced coronary constriction was demonstrated in female patients receiving continuous physiological concentrations of intracoronary 17β-oestradiol (Gilligan et al, 1994b).

The response of coronary arteries to acetylcholine after exposure to 17β-oestradiol is gender-dependent (Figure 7) (Collins et al, 1995). 17β-Oestradiol modulates acetylcholine-induced coronary artery responses of female but not male atherosclerotic coronary arteries in vivo. These human data confirm reports from studies in cynomolgus monkeys that oestrogen modulates the responses of atherosclerotic coronary arteries. An enhancement of endothelium-dependent relaxation by natural oestrogen (as used in most HRT) may be important in post-menopausal women with established CHD and may contribute to the acute effect of 17β-oestradiol on blood flow and its long-term protective effect on the development of coronary artery disease. The mechanisms of this in vivo response are not well understood but could be due to a number of synergistic mechanisms, such as enhanced endothelium-dependent relaxation. Inhibition of constrictor responses to endothelin-I (Jiang et al, 1992c) and angiotensin-II (Ravi et al, 1994) may

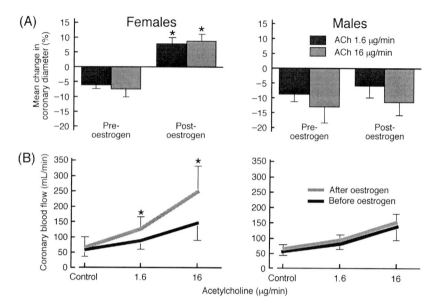

Figure 7. (A) Mean change in diameter of coronary artery in females and males evoked by acetyl-choline (ACh) before and after oestrogen (* $P < 0.01$ pre- versus post-oestrogen) ▪, ACh 1.6 µg/min; ▨, 16 µg/min). (B) Coronary blood flow increase in females and males before and after oestrogen (* $P < 0.009$ pre- versus post-oestrogen).

also contribute to the net reversal of acetylcholine-induced coronary constriction. In contrast, conjugated equine oestrogen has been shown to improve vascular reactivity in male rhesus monkeys (Wagner et al, 1995) and humans (Blumenthal et al, 1996), however this effect may be dose-dependent.

Prostaglandins

Prostacyclin (PGI_2) is a prostaglandin produced by the endothelial cells. Its synthesis is thought to be coupled to EDRF release (Botting and Vane, 1989), and it can induce vasodilatation and inhibit platelet activation. Oestrogen can upregulate the production of prostacyclin (Mendelsohn and Karas, 1994). Chang et al (1980) demonstrated an enhancement of basal levels of prostacyclin secretion in rat aortic smooth muscle cells exposed to oestradiol. This was thought to be mediated via a receptor-dependent mechanism stimulating the enzymes prostacyclin synthetase and prostaglandin cyclooxygenase. The evidence is scant however, and has yet to be demonstrated in human tissue, but there is an indication that oestrogen may affect coagulation and vasorelaxation by its effects on prostacyclin.

Inhibition of atherogenesis

The benefits of ORT on CVD risk may be partially explained by oestrogen-associated reduction in LDL-C and increase in HDL-C (Knopp, 1988), and this in turn will affect the progression of atheroma development. Animal studies show that long-term oestrogen replacement inhibits the progression of atherosclerosis, reducing plaque size (Adams et al, 1990). 17β-Oestradiol plus cyclical progestogen treatment for 18 weeks in ovariectomized cynomolgus monkeys showed a decreased accumulation of LDL-C in the coronary arteries compared to non-treated controls, with no effect on plasma lipid, lipoprotein or apoprotein concentrations, nor endothelial cell turnover or leukocyte adhesion. Arterial intimal lesions were no different between groups (Wagner et al, 1991). They concluded that sex hormones inhibit the initiation of atheroma deposition by a direct effect at the arterial wall, either decreasing LDL-C uptake and/or its degradation. Chronic stress induced by subordination has been shown to result in impaired ovarian function in premenopausal female monkeys (Kaplan et al, 1984). These animals also had decreased HDL cholesterol levels and more atherosclerosis than dominant animals, suggesting that the disturbance of ovarian function may adversely affect atheroma formation by its effects on lipid profile (Figure 8).

Retrospective angiographic studies support an apparent protective effect of oestrogen on atheroma progression in humans. Oestrogen users have less coronary artery occlusion compared to non-users (Gruchow et al, 1988), and less angiographically significant coronary artery disease (Sullivan et al,

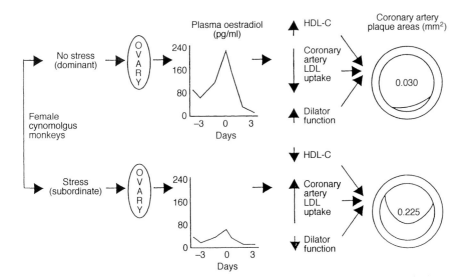

Figure 8. Disturbance of ovarian function in chronically stressed animals may affect the atherosclerotic process by affecting lipid profile. Adapted from Clarkson et al (1994).

1988). This effect of oestrogen was independent of type of menopause or other cardiovascular risk factors, except HDL-C.

Thus, long-term HRT appears to affect atheroma initiation and progression. The mechanism may be via the classical oestrogen receptor, but numerous factors seem to be involved and their role in vascular regulation still needs to be clarified (Figure 9).

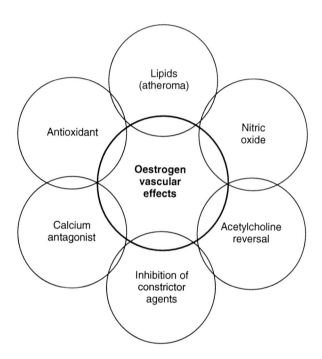

Figure 9. Some of the potential mechanisms involved in the direct vascular effects of oestrogen. A synergistic interaction between these mechanisms is likely.

Progestogens

Much of the data reported has been with oestrogen alone treatment. This may be misleading clinically since many women taking HRT are on a progestogen combined with oestrogen which protects against endometrial cancer. Progesterone is an antagonist of oestrogen in the reproductive system, therefore it is assumed that the addition of a progestogen may oppose the beneficial effects of oestrogen on the cardiovascular system. Epidemiological studies have investigated the effect of the addition of a progestogen to oestrogen therapy on cardiovascular morbidity and mortality. A recent study has shown that a progestin added to oestrogen therapy does not alter the cardioprotective effect of postmenopausal oestrogen use (Grodstein et al, 1996).

The effect of progestogen on serum lipids is dependent on the type and dose used. In usual therapeutic doses, 19-nortestosterone compounds decrease both HDL-C and triglycerides, and 17-hydroxyprogestins have little effect on lipids. Progestogens increase hepatic lipase activity, increasing catabolism of HDL_2 and thereby decreasing plasma levels of HDL_2 and HDL-C (Tikkanen et al, 1986). There is no effect on LDL-C levels. However, in combination with oestrogen, observational studies have demonstrated a nil or beneficial effect of progestogens on lipid profile. Nabulsi et al (1993) found a more favourable lipid and coagulation profile with combination therapy. Adams et al (1990) found no effect of progestogen on the beneficial effect of ORT in ovariectomized cynomolgus monkeys with coronary artery atherosclerosis on long-term treatment. There was also no difference between groups in lipid profile.

The effect of the addition of a progestogen on insulin resistance depends on the androgenicity of the progestogen used—non-androgenic progestogens, including norethindrone acetate (Godsland et al, 1993) and dydrogesterone (Stevenson et al, 1994), tend not to oppose the oestrogen-induced benefits on insulin sensitivity. The method of administration also appears to be important, with oral combined HRT (norgestrel) having a negative effect on insulin resistance, and transdermal therapy (norethisterone) having little or no effect.

Progesterone relaxes (Jiang et al, 1992b) rabbit coronary arteries in vitro by an endothelium-independent mechanism, indicating that progesterone may have different effects on the circulation of reproductive and other organs. Coronary artery relaxation was examined in ovariectomized dogs treated with oestrogen, progestogen, or oestrogen plus progestogen therapy (Miller and Vanhoutte, 1991). While progesterone alone minimally affected endothelium-dependent responses, the relaxation response to acetylcholine was less in the combined oestrogen plus progestogen group than the oestrogen alone group. The conclusion was that progestogen antagonizes the stimulatory effect of oestrogen on the production of NO. A similar study has yet to be reported in humans.

CEREBROVASCULAR CIRCULATION

Oestrogen status affects the reactivity of cerebral arteries to vasoactive stimuli such as serotonin. Using hormone manipulation in rabbits, oestrogen withdrawal selectively increased serotonin reactivity in rabbit basilar arteries (Shay et al, 1994). Basilar artery segments from chronically oophorectomized animals treated with oestrogen, which were subsequently acutely oestrogen withdrawn, showed an extremely heightened sensitivity to the vasoconstrictor response to serotonin. This state may be similar to post-menopausal women on HRT who sustain acute oestrogen withdrawal, or the perimenopausal state associated with oestrogen surges.

Vascular reactivity changes in the central retinal and ophthalmic arteries can be correlated with oestrogen status in pregnant and post-menopausal women (Belfort et al, 1995). There are also gender differences in cerebral blood flow related to oestrogen. Until the menopause, cerebral blood flow is greater in women than men of the same age (Shaw et al, 1984), however after the menopause, cerebral blood flow decreases in females and is the same as age-matched males (Rodriguez et al, 1988). ORT in post-menopausal women reduces resistance in the internal carotid (Ganger et al, 1991; Penotti et al, 1993) and middle cerebral arteries (Penotti et al, 1993). Cerebral blood flow is also increased in pregnancy when oestrogen levels are substantially increased (Ikeda et al, 1993). Velocity changes in the middle cerebral artery have been studied during controlled ovarian hyper-stimulation after pituitary suppression (Shamma et al, 1992). Oestrogen levels directly correlated with middle cerebral artery velocity and resist-ance. It was hypothesized that there was microcirculatory dilatation distal to the middle cerebral artery. Oestrogenic effects have recently been identified in smaller vessels such as the central retinal artery (Belfort et al, 1995).

HRT in women, either in established menopause or in the peri-menopause, is associated with a decreased risk of cerebrovascular accident (Ross et al, 1989). In older women (aged ≥ 75 years), ORT may decrease the risk of stroke by up to 50% (Paganini-Hill et al, 1988). Ever users of post-menopausal HRT have a greater decrease in risk of stroke than never users (Finucane et al, 1993) and current use is more protective than ever use (Falkeborn et al, 1993).

SUMMARY

Combining the wealth of epidemiological, metabolic and recent mech-anistic data, it would appear biologically plausible that HRT, either oestrogen alone or in combination with progestogen, is cardioprotective. Further research is required, as information is lacking on cardiovascular effects of HRT instigated at an older age. There is a need to identify cardio-vascular benefit, indirect and/or direct, of combined oestrogen/progestogen therapy using randomized trials. The various progestogen types and doses also need to be investigated. Studies are also required to investigate the effect of HRT use in higher risk patients with established CVD. There is scant information on the effect of HRT on blood pressure of patients with hypertension.

Cardiovascular risk factor profiles and incidence surveys need to be conducted in developing countries to characterize their female population and to identify the prevalence of CVD; this needs to be undertaken before widespread recommendations on CVD prevention and the role of HRT can be made.

If HRT is to be used effectively in the future treatment of heart disease in women these questions need to be addressed. At present HRT is indi-cated for the relief of menopausal symptoms and the prevention of osteo-porosis. In women without these indications, ORT may be recommended in those who have had a premature menopause, and possibly in those who have established CHD or who are at high risk of developing CHD. It is too early to suggest a blanket recommendation for the use of HRT in the treatment of the symptoms of women with established CVD, but HRT after the menopause may at least be safely used in the secondary prevention of CHD.

REFERENCES

Abbott WG, Lillioja S, Young AA et al (1987) Relationships between plasma lipoprotein concentrations and insulin action in an obese hyperinsulinemic population. *Diabetes* **36:** 897–904.

Adam S, Williams V & Vessey MP (1981) Cardiovascular disease and hormone replacement treatment: a pilot case-control study. *British Medical Journal* **282:** 1277–1278.

Adams MR, Kaplan JR, Manuck SB et al (1990) Inhibition of coronary artery atherosclerosis by 17-beta estradiol in ovariectomized monkeys. Lack of an effect of added progesterone. *Arteriosclerosis* **10:** 1051–1057.

Anonymous (1995) Effects of estrogen or estrogen/progestin regimens on heart disease risk factors in postmenopausal women. The Postmenopausal Estrogen/Progestin Interventions (PEPI) Trial. The Writing Group for the PEPI Trial. *Journal of the American Medical Association* **273:** 199–208.

Bain C, Willett W, Hennekens CH et al (1981) Use of postmenopausal hormones and risk of myocardial infarction. *Circulation* **64:** 42–46.

Barrett-Connor E, Wingard DL & Criqui MH (1989) Postmenopausal estrogen use and heart disease risk factors in the 1980s. Rancho Bernardo, Calif, revisited. *Journal of the American Medical Association* **261:** 2095–2100.

Barrett-Connor E & Bush TL (1991) Estrogen and coronary heart disease in women. *Journal of the American Medical Association* **265:** 1861–1867.

Belfort MA, Saade GR, Snabes M et al (1995) Hormonal status affects the reactivity of the cerebral vasculature. *American Journal of Obstetrics and Gynecology* **172:** 1273–1278.

Blumenthal RS, Gloth ST, Reis SE et al (1996) Acute administration of estrogen improves coronary vasomotor response to acetylcholine in men. *Journal of the American College of Cardiology* **27(2):** 287A.

Botting R & Vane JR (1989) The receipt and dispatch of chemical messengers by endothelial cells. In Schrör K & Sinzinger H (eds) *Prostaglandins in Clinical Research: Cardiovascular System*, pp 1–11. New York: Alan R. Liss.

Brezinka V & Padmos I (1994) Coronary heart disease risk factors in women. *European Heart Journal* **15:** 1571–1584.

Burch JC, Byrd BF Jr & Vaughn WK (1974) The effects of long-term estrogen on hysterectomized women. *American Journal of Obstetrics and Gynecology* **118:** 778–782.

Bush TL, Barrett-Connor E, Cowan LD et al (1987) Cardiovascular mortality and noncontraceptive use of estrogen in women: results from the Lipid Research Clinics Program Follow-up Study. *Circulation* **75:** 1102–1109.

Byrd BF Jr, Burch JC & Vaughn WK (1977) The impact of long term estrogen support after hysterectomy. A report of 1016 cases. *Annals of Surgery* **185:** 574–580.

Cagnacci A, Soldani R, Carriero PL et al (1992) Effects of low doses of transdermal 17 beta-estradiol on carbohydrate metabolism in postmenopausal women. *Journal of Clinical Endocrinology and Metabolism* **74:** 1396–1400.

Cannon RO & Epstein SE (1988) 'Microvascular angina' as a cause of chest pain with angiographically normal coronary arteries. *American Journal of Cardiology* **61:** 1338–1343.

Caulin-Glaser TL, Sessa W, Sarrel P & Bender J (1994) The effect of 17β-estradiol on human endothelial cell nitric oxide production. *Circulation* **90:** I-30.

Chang WC, Nakao J, Orimo H & Murota S (1980) Stimulation of prostacyclin biosynthetic activity by estradiol in rat aortic smooth muscle cells in culture. *Biochemica et Biophysica Acta* **619:** 107–118.

Chester AH, Jiang C, Borland JA et al (1995) Estrogen relaxes human epicardial coronary arteries through non-endothelium-dependent mechanisms. *Coronary Artery Disease* **6:** 417–422.

Clarke KW, Gray D, Keating NA & Hampton JR (1994) Do women with acute myocardial infarction receive the same treatment as men? [see comments]. *British Medical Journal* **309**: 563–566.

Clarkson TB (1994) Estrogen, progestins, and coronary heart disease in cynomolgus monkeys. *Fertility and Sterility* **62(6) supplement 2:** 147S–151S.

Clarkson TB, Anthony MS & Potvin-Klein K (1994) Effects of estrogen treatment on arterial wall structure and function. *Drugs* **47 (supplement 2):** 42–51.

Colditz GA, Willett WC, Stampfer MJ et al (1987) Menopause and the risk of coronary heart disease in women. *New England Journal of Medicine* **316:** 1105–1110.

Collins P, Rosano GMC, Jiang C et al (1993) Hypothesis: Cardiovascular protection by oestrogen—a calcium antagonist effect? *Lancet* **341:** 1264–1265.

Collins P, Shay J, Jiang C & Moss J (1994) Nitric oxide accounts for dose-dependent estrogen--mediated coronary relaxation following acute estrogen withdrawal. *Circulation* **90:** 1964–1968.

Collins P, Rosano GMC, Sarrel PM et al (1995) Estradiol-17β attenuates acetylcholine-induced coronary arterial constriction in women but not men with coronary heart disease. *Circulation* **92:** 24–30.

Criqui MH, Suarez L, Barrett-Connor E et al (1988) Postmenopausal estrogen use and mortality. Results from a prospective study in a defined, homogeneous community. *American Journal of Epidemiology* **128:** 606–614.

Croft P & Hannaford P (1989a) Risk factors for acute myocardial infarction in women: evidence from the Royal College of General Practitioners' oral contraceptive study. *Cardiovascular Medicine* **8:** 71.

Croft P & Hannaford PC (1989b) Risk factors for acute myocardial infarction in women: evidence from the Royal College of General Practitioners' oral contraception study. *British Medical Journal* **298:** 165–168.

Dubey RK & Overbeck HW (1994) Culture of rat mesenteric arteriolar smooth muscle cells: effects of platelet-derived growth factor, angiotensin, and nitric oxide on growth. *Cell Tissue Research* **275:** 133–141.

Eaker E, Chesebro JH, Sacks FM et al (1993) Cardiovascular disease in women. *Circulation* **88:** 1999–2009.

Falkeborn M, Persson I, Adami HO et al (1992) The risk of acute myocardial infarction after oestrogen and oestrogen-progestogen replacement. *British Journal of Obstetrics and Gynaecology* **99:** 821–828.

Falkeborn M, Persson I, Terent A et al (1993) Hormone replacement therapy and the risk of stroke. Follow-up of a population-based cohort in Sweden. *Archives of Internal Medicine* **153:** 1201–1209.

Finucane FF, Madans JH, Bush TL et al (1993) Decreased risk of stroke among postmenopausal hormone users. Results from a national cohort. *Archives of Internal Medicine* **153:** 73–79.

Folsom AR, Wu KK, Davis CE et al (1991) Population correlates of plasma fibrinogen and factor VII, putative cardiovascular risk factors. *Atherosclerosis* **91:** 191–205.

Ganger KF, Vyas S, Whitehead M et al (1991) Pulsatility index in internal carotid artery in relation to transdermal oestradiol and time since menopause. *Lancet* **338:** 839–842.

Gebara OCE, Mittleman MA, Sutherland P et al (1995) Association between increased estrogen status and increased fibrinolytic potential in the Framingham Offspring study. *Circulation* **91:** 1952–1958.

Gilligan DM, Badar DM, Panza JA et al (1994a) Acute vascular effects of estrogen in postmenopausal women. *Circulation* **90:** 786–791.

Gilligan DM, Quyyumi AA & Cannon RO, III (1994b) Effects of physiological levels of estrogen on coronary vasomotor function in postmenopausal women. *Circulation* **89:** 2545–2551.

Ginsburg J & Hardiman P (1989) The peripheral circulation in the menopause. In Ginsburg J (eds) *The Circulation in the Female*, pp 99–115. Carnforth: Parthenon.

Godsland IF, Wynn V, Crook D & Miller NE (1987) Sex, plasma lipoproteins, and atherosclerosis: prevailing assumptions and outstanding questions. *American Heart Journal* **114:** 1467–1503.

Godsland IF, Gangar KF, Walton C et al (1993) Insulin resistance, secretion, and elimination in post-menopausal women receiving oral or transdermal hormone replacement therapy. *Metabolism* **42:** 846–853.

Gordon T, Kannel WB, Hjortland MC & Mcnamara PM (1978) Menopause and coronary heart disease. The Framingham Study. *Annals of Internal Medicine* **89:** 157–161.

Grady D, Rubin SM, Petitti DB et al (1992) Hormone therapy to prevent disease and prolong life in postmenopausal women. *Annals of Internal Medicine* **117:** 1016–1037.

Grodstein F, Stampfer MJ, Manson J et al (1996) Postmenopausal estrogen and progestin use and the risk of cardiovascular disease. *New England Journal of Medicine* **335:** 453–461.

Gruchow HW, Anderson AJ, Barboriak JJ & Sobocinski KA (1988) Postmenopausal use of estrogen and occlusion of coronary arteries. *American Heart Journal* **115:** 954–963.

Hammond CB, Jelovsek FR, Lee KL et al (1979) Effects of long-term estrogen replacement therapy. I. Metabolic effects. *American Journal of Obstetrics and Gynecology* **133:** 525–536.

Han SZ, Karaki H, Ouchi Y et al (1995) 17β-Estradiol inhibits Ca2+ influx and Ca2+ release induced by thromboxane A2 in porcine coronary artery. *Circulation* **91:** 2619–2626.

Hayashi T, Fukuto JM, Ignarro LJ & Chaudhuri G (1992) Basal release of nitric oxide from aortic rings is greater in female rabbits than in male rabbits: implications for atherosclerosis. *Proceedings of the National Academy of Sciences of the United States of America* **89:** 11 259–11 263.

Hazzard WR (1989) Estrogen replacement and cardiovascular disease: serum lipids and blood pressure effects. *American Journal of Obstetrics and Gynecology* **161:** 1847–1853.

Heinrich J, Sandkamp M, Kokott R et al (1991) Relationship of lipoprotein(a) to variables of coagulation and fibrinolysis in a healthy population. *Clinical Chemistry* **37:** 1950–1954.

Hemminki E & Sihvo S (1993) A review of postmenopausal hormone therapy recommendations: potential for selection bias. *Obstetrics and Gynecology* **82:** 1021–1028.

Henderson BE, Ross RK, Paganini-Hill A & Mack TM (1986) Estrogen use and cardiovascular disease. *American Journal of Obstetrics and Gynecology* **154:** 1181–1186.

Henderson BE, Paganini-Hill A & Ross RK (1988) Estrogen replacement therapy and protection from acute myocardial infarction. *American Journal of Obstetrics and Gynecology* **159:** 312–317.

Henderson BE, Paginini-Hill A & Rossk RK (1991) Decreased mortality in users of estrogen replacement therapy. *Archives of Internal Medicine* **151:** 75–78.

Hunt K, Vessey M & McPherson K (1990) Mortality in a cohort of long-term users of hormone replacement therapy: an updated analysis. *British Journal of Obstetrics and Gynaecology* **97:** 1080–1086.

Ikeda T, Ikenoue T, Mori N et al (1993) Effect of early pregnancy on maternal regional cerebral blood flow. *American Journal of Obstetrics and Gynecology* **168:** 1303–1308.

Jiang C, Sarrel PM, Lindsay DC et al (1991) Endothelium-independent relaxation of rabbit coronary artery by 17β-oestradiol in vitro. *British Journal of Pharmacology* **104:** 1033–1037.

Jiang C, Poole-Wilson PA, Sarrel PM et al (1992a) Effect of 17β-oestradiol on contraction, Ca^{2+} current and intracellular free Ca^{2+} in guinea-pig isolated cardiac myocytes. *British Journal of Pharmacology* **106:** 739–745.

Jiang C, Sarrel PM, Lindsay DC et al (1992b) Progesterone induces endothelium-independent relaxation of rabbit coronary artery in vitro. *European Journal of Pharmacology* **211:** 163–167.

Jiang C, Sarrel PM, Poole-Wilson PA & Collins P (1992c) Acute effect of 17β-estradiol on rabbit coronary artery contractile responses to endothelin-1. *American Journal of Physiology* **263:** H271–H275.

Jick H, Dinan B & Rothman KJ (1978) Noncontraceptive estrogens and nonfatal myocardial infarction. *Journal of the American Medical Association* **239:** 1407–1409.

Kaplan JR, Adams MR, Clarkson TB & Koritnik DR (1984) Psychosocial influences on female 'protection' among cynomolgus macaques. *Atherosclerosis* **53:** 283–295.

Kaski JC, Rosano GMC, Collins P et al (1995) Cardiac syndrome X: clinical characteristics and left ventricular function. Long term follow-up study. *Journal of the American College of Cardiology* **25:** 807–814.

Kemp HG, Jr, Vokonas PS, Cohn PF & Gorlin R (1973) The anginal syndrome associated with normal coronary arteriograms. Report of a six year experience. *American Journal of Medicine* **54:** 735–742.

Knopp RH (1988) The effects of postmenopausal estrogen therapy on the incidence of arteriosclerotic vascular disease. *Obstetrics and Gynecology* **72:** 23S–30S.

Kronenberg F, Cote LJ, Linkie DM et al (1984) Menopausal hot flushes: thermoregulatory, cardiovascular and circulating catecholamine and LH changes. *Maturitas* **6:** 31–43.

Lafferty FW & Fiske ME (1994) Postmenopausal estrogen replacement: a long-term cohort study. *American Journal of Medicine* **97:** 66–77.

Lafferty FW & Helmuth DO (1985) Post-menopausal estrogen replacement: the prevention of osteoporosis and systemic effects. *Maturitas* **7:** 147–159.

Lichtlen PR, Hugenholtz PG, Rafflenbeul W et al (1990) Retardation of angiographic progression of coronary artery disease by nifedipine. *Lancet* **335:** 1109–1113.

Likoff W, Segal BL & Kasparian H (1967) Paradox of normal selective coronary arteriograms in patients considered to have unmistakable coronary heart disease. *New England Journal of Medicine* **276:** 1063–1066.

Lind T, Cameron EC, Hunter WM et al (1979) A prospective, controlled trial of six forms of hormone replacement therapy given to postmenopausal women. *British Journal of Obstetrics and Gynaecology* **86 (supplement 3):** 1–29.

Lip G, Beevers M, Holmes A et al (1994) Effects of hormone replacement therapy (HRT) on blood pressure in hypertensive women. *Journal of the American College of Cardiology* 348A.

Lip GY, Beevers G & Zarifis J (1995) Hormone replacement therapy and cardiovascular risk: the cardiovascular physicians' viewpoint. *Journal of Internal Medicine* **238:** 389.

Lobo RA (1991) Clinical review 27: Effects of hormonal replacement on lipids and lipoproteins in postmenopausal women. *Journal of Clinical Endocrinology and Metabolism* **73:** 925–930.

Luotola H (1983) Blood pressure and hemodynamics in postmenopausal women during estradiol-17 beta substitution. *Annals of Clinical Research* **15 (supplement 38):** 1–121.

McFarland KF, Boniface ME, Hornung CA et al (1989) Risk factors and noncontraceptive estrogen use in women with and without coronary disease. *American Heart Journal* **117:** 1209–1214.

Magness RR, Rosenfeld CR, Faucher DJ & Mitchell MD (1992) Uterine prostaglandin production in ovine pregnancy: effects of angiotensin II and indomethacin. *American Journal of Physiology* **263:** H188–H197.

Magness RR & Rosenfeld CR (1989) Local and systemic estradiol-17 beta: effects on uterine and systemic vasodilation. *American Journal of Physiology* **256:** E536–E542.

Manolio TA, Furberg CD, Shemanski L et al (1993) Associations of postmenopausal estrogen use with cardiovascular disease and its risk factors in older women. The CHS Collaborative Research Group. *Circulation* **88:** 2163–2171.

Maseri A, Crea F, Kaski JC & Crake T (1991) Mechanisms of angina pectoris in syndrome X. *Journal of the American College of Cardiology* **17:** 499–506.

Mendelsohn ME & Karas RH (1994) Estrogen and the blood vessel wall. *Current Opinion in Cardiology* **9:** 619–626.

Miller VM & Vanhoutte PM (1991) Progesterone and modulation of endothelium-dependent responses in canine coronary arteries. *American Journal of Physiology* **261:** R1022–R1027.

MRC Working Party (1992) Medical Research Council trial of treatment of hypertension in older adults: principal results. *British Medical Journal* **304:** 405–412.

Muck AO, Seeger H, Korte K & Lippert TH (1993) The effect of 17 beta-estradiol and endothelin 1 on prostacyclin and thromboxane production in human endothelial cell cultures. *Clinical and Experimental Obstetrics and Gynecology* **20:** 203–206.

Mügge A, Riedel M, Barton M et al (1993) Endothelium independent relaxation of human coronary arteries by 17beta-oestradiol in vitro. *Cardiovascular Research* **27:** 1939–1942.

Myers PR, Guerra RJ & Harrison DG (1989) Release of NO and EDRF from cultured bovine aortic endothelial cells. *American Journal of Physiology* **256:** H1030–H1037.

Nabulsi AA, Folsom AR, White A et al (1993) Association of hormone-replacement therapy with various cardiovascular risk factors in postmenopausal women. The Atherosclerosis Risk in Communities Study Investigators. *New England Journal of Medicine* **328:** 1069–1075.

Nachtigall LE, Nachtigall RH, Nachtigall RD & Beckman EM (1979) Estrogen replacement therapy II: a prospective study in the relationship to carcinoma and cardiovascular and metabolic problems. *Obstetrics and Gynecology* **54:** 74–79.

Opherk D, Zebe H, Weihe E et al (1981) Reduced coronary dilatory capacity and ultrastructural changes of the myocardium in patients with angina pectoris but normal coronary arteriograms. *Circulation* **63:** 817–825.

Paganini-Hill A, Ross RK & Henderson BE (1988) Postmenopausal oestrogen treatment and stroke: a prospective study. *British Medical Journal* **297:** 519–522.

Palmer RM, Ferrige AG & Moncada S (1987) Nitric oxide release accounts for the biological activity of endothelium-derived relaxing factor. *Nature* **327:** 524–526.

Penotti M, Nencioni T, Gabrielli L et al (1993) Blood flow variations in internal carotid and middle cerebral arteries induced by postmenopausal hormone replacement therapy. *American Journal of Obstetrics and Gynecology* **169:** 1226–1232.

Peters NS, Rosano GMC, Sarrel P et al (1994) A randomised double-blind crossover placebo-controlled trial of oestradiol-17β therapy in female patients with syndrome X. *European Heart Journal* **15:** 10.

Petitti DB, Perlman JA & Sidney S (1987) Noncontraceptive estrogens and mortality: long-term follow-up of women in the Walnut Creek Study. *Obstetrics and Gynecology* **70:** 289–293.

Pfeffer RI & van den Noort S (1976) Estrogen use and stroke risk in postmenopausal women. *American Journal of Epidemiology* **103:** 445–456.

Pfeffer RI, Whipple GH, Kurosaki TT & Chapman JM (1978) Coronary risk and estrogen use in post-menopausal women. *American Journal of Epidemiology* **107:** 479–497.

Pfeffer RI, Kurosaki TT & Charlton SK (1979) Estrogen use and blood pressure in later life. *American Journal of Epidemiology* **110:** 469–478.

Phibbs B, Fleming T, Ewy GA et al (1988) Frequency of normal coronary arteriograms in three academic medical centers and one community hospital. *American Journal of Cardiology* **62:** 472–474.

Pines A, Fisman EZ, Levo Y et al (1991) The effects of hormone replacement therapy in normal post-menopausal women: measurements of Doppler-derived parameters of aortic flow. *American Journal of Obstetrics and Gynecology* **164:** 806–812.

Pines A, Fisman EZ, Drory Y et al (1992) Menopause-induced changes in doppler-derived parameters of aortic flow in healthy women. *American Journal of Cardiology* **69:** 1104–1106.

Pinto S, Rostagno C, Coppo M et al (1990) No signs of increased thrombin generation in menopause. *Thrombosis Research* **58:** 645–651.

Polderman KH, Stehouwer CDA, van Kamp GJ et al (1993) Influence of sex hormones on plasma endothelin levels. *Annals of Internal Medicine* **118:** 429–432.

Psaty BM, Heckbert SR, Atkins D et al (1994) The risk of myocardial infarction associated with the combined use of estrogens and progestins in postmenopausal women. *Archives of Internal Medicine* **154:** 1333–1339.

Ravi J, Mantzoros CS, Prabhu AS et al (1994) In vitro relaxation of phenylephrine- and angiotensin II-contracted aortic rings by beta-estradiol. *American Journal of Hypertension* **7:** 1065–1069.

Rees MC & Barlow DH (1988) Absence of sustained reflex vasoconstriction in women with menopausal flushes. *Human Reproduction* **3:** 823–825.

Reis SE, Gloth ST, Blumenthal RS et al (1994) Ethinyl estradiol acutely attenuates abnormal coronary vasomotor responses to acetylcholine in postmenopausal women. *Circulation* **89:** 52–60.

Rich-Edwards JW, Manson JE, Hennekens CH & Buring JE (1995) The primary prevention of coronary heart disease in women. *New England Journal of Medicine* **332:** 1758–1766.

Rodriguez G, Warkentin S, Risberg J & Rosadini G (1988) Sex differences in regional cerebral blood flow. *Journal of Cerebral Blood Flow Metabolism* **8:** 783–789.

Rosano GMC, Lindsay DC & Poole-Wilson PA (1991) Syndrome X: an hypothesis for cardiac pain without ischaemia. *Cardiologia* **36:** 885–895.

Rosano GMC, Collins P, Kaski JC et al (1995) Syndrome X in women is associated with estrogen deficiency. *European Heart Journal* **16:** 610–614.

Rosano GMC, Peters NS, Lefroy D et al (1996) 17β-Estradiol therapy improves angina in post-menopausal women with syndrome X. *Journal of the American College of Cardiology* (in press).

Rose GA & Blackburn H (1968) *Cardiovascular Survey Methods*, Geneva: World Health Organization Monograph Series Number 56.

Rosenberg L, Armstrong B & Jick H (1976) Myocardial infarction and estrogen therapy in post-menopausal women. *New England Journal of Medicine* **294:** 1256–1259.

Rosenberg L, Palmer JR & Shapiro S (1990) Decline in the risk of myocardial infarction among women who stop smoking. *New England Journal of Medicine* **322:** 213–217.

Rosenberg SH, Fausone V & Clark R (1980) The role of estrogens as a risk factor for stroke in post-menopausal women. *Western Journal of Medicine* **133:** 292–296.

Ross RK, Paganini-Hill A, Mack TM et al (1981) Menopausal oestrogen therapy and protection from death from ischaemic heart disease. *Lancet* **1:** 858–860.

Ross RK, Pike MC, Henderson BE et al (1989) Stroke prevention and oestrogen replacement therapy. *Lancet* **March 4:** 505.

Sack MN, Rader DJ & Cannon RO, III (1994) Oestrogen and inhibition of oxidation of low-density lipoproteins in postmenopausal women. *Lancet* **343:** 269–270.

Scarabin PY, Bonithon-Kopp C, Bara L et al (1990) Factor VII activation and menopausal status. *Thrombosis Research* **57:** 227–234.

Schray-Utz B, Zeiher AM & Busse R (1993) Expression of constitutive NO synthase in cultured endothelial cells is enhanced by 17β-estradiol. *Circulation* **88:** 1–80.

Shamma FN, Fayad P, Brass L & Sarrel P (1992) Middle cerebral artery blood velocity during controlled ovarian hyperstimulation. *Fertility and Sterility* **57:** 1022–1025.

Shaw TG, Mortel KF, Meyer JS et al (1984) Cerebral blood flow changes in benign aging and cerebrovascular disease. *Neurology* **34:** 855–862.

Shay J, Futo J, Badrov N & Moss J (1994) Estrogen withdrawal selectively increases serotonin reactivity in rabbit basilar artery. *Life Sciences* **55:** 1071–1081.

Shively CA & Clarkson TB (1994) Social status and coronary artery atherosclerosis in female monkeys. *Arteriosclerosis and Thrombosis* **14(5):** 721–726.

Simon BC, Cunningham LD & Cohen RA (1990) Oxidized low density lipoproteins cause contraction and inhibit endothelium-dependent relaxation in the pig coronary artery. *Journal of Clinical Investigation* **86:** 75–79.

Soma M, Fumagalli R, Paoletti R et al (1991) Plasma Lp(a) concentration after oestrogen and progestagen in postmenopausal women. *Lancet* **337:** 612.

Stampfer MJ & Colditz GA (1991) Estrogen replacement therapy and coronary heart disease: a quantitative assessment of the epidemiologic evidence. *Preventive Medicine* **20:** 47–63.

Stampfer MJ, Willett WC, Colditz GA et al (1985) A prospective study of postmenopausal estrogen therapy and coronary heart disease. *New England Journal of Medicine* **313:** 1044–1049.

Stampfer MJ, Colditz GA, Willett WC et al (1991) Postmenopausal estrogen therapy and cardiovascular disease. *New England Journal of Medicine* **325:** 756–762.

Steingart RM, Packer M, Hamm P et al (1991) Sex differences in the management of coronary artery disease. Survival and Ventricular Enlargement Investigators. *New England Journal of Medicine* **325:** 226–230.

Stevenson JC, Crook D & Godsland IF (1993) Influence of age and menopause on serum lipids and lipoproteins in healthy women. *Atherosclerosis* **98:** 83–90.

Stevenson JC, Crook D, Godsland IF et al (1994) Hormone replacement therapy and the cardiovascular system nonlipid effects. *Drugs* **47 (supplement 2):** 35–41.

Sullivan JM, Vander Zwaag R, Lemp GF et al (1988) Postmenopausal estrogen use and coronary atherosclerosis. *Annals of Internal Medicine* **108:** 358–363.

Sullivan JM, Vander Zwaag R, Hughes JP et al (1990) Estrogen replacement and coronary artery disease. Effect on survival in postmenopausal women. *Archives of Internal Medicine* **150:** 2557–2562.

Szklo M, Tonascia J, Gordis L & Bloom I (1984) Estrogen use and myocardial infarction risk: a case-control study. *Preventive Medicine* **13:** 510–516.

Tikkanen MJ, Kuusi T, Nikkila EA & Sipinen S (1986) Post-menopausal hormone replacement therapy: effects of progestogens on serum lipids and lipoproteins. A review. *Maturitas* **8:** 7–17.

Turiel M, Galassi AR, Glazier JJ et al (1987) Pain threshold and tolerance in women with syndrome X and women with stable angina pectoris. *American Journal of Cardiology* **60:** 503–507.

Van Buren G, Yang D & Clark KE (1992) Estrogen-induced uterine vasodilatation is antagonized by L-nitroarginine methyl ester, an inhibitor of nitric oxide synthesis. *American Journal of Obstetrics and Gynecology* **16:** 828–833.

Volterrani M, Rosano GMC, Coats A et al (1995) Estrogen acutely increases peripheral blood flow in postmenopausal women. *American Journal of Medicine* **99:** 119–122.

Wagner JD, Clarkson TB, St Clair RW et al (1991) Estrogen and progesterone replacement therapy reduces low density lipoprotein accumulation in the coronary arteries of surgically postmenopausal cynomolgus monkeys. *Journal of Clinical Investigation* **88:** 1995–2002.

Wagner JD, Washburn SA, Zhang L et al (1995) A non-feminizing conjugated equine estrogen decreases arterial LDL degradation and improves vascular reactivity in male rhesus monkeys. *Circulation* **92:** I-627.

Walsh BW, Schiff I, Rosner B et al (1991) Effects of postmenopausal estrogen replacement on the concentrations and metabolism of plasma lipoproteins. *New England Journal of Medicine* **325:** 1196–1204.

Waters D, Lesperance J, Francetich M et al (1990) A controlled clinical trial to assess the effect of a calcium channel blocker on the progression of coronary atherosclerosis. *Circulation* **82:** 1940–1953.

Weiner CP, Lizasoain I, Baylis SA et al (1994) Induction of calcium-dependent nitric oxide synthases by sex hormones. *Proceedings of the National Academy of Sciences of the United States of America* **91:** 5212–5216.

Williams JK, Adams MR & Klopfenstein HS (1990) Estrogen modulates responses of atherosclerotic coronary arteries. *Circulation* **81:** 1680–1687.

Williams JK, Adams MR, Herrington DM & Clarkson TB (1992) Short-term administration of estrogen and vascular responses of atherosclerotic coronary arteries. *Journal of the American College of Cardiology* **20:** 452–457.

Williams JK, Honore EK, Washburn SA & Clarkson TB (1994) Effects of hormone replacement therapy on reactivity of atherosclerotic coronary arteries in cynomolgus monkeys. *Journal of the American College of Cardiology* **24:** 1757–1761.

Wilson PW, Garrison RJ & Castelli WP (1985) Postmenopausal estrogen use, cigarette smoking, and cardiovascular morbidity in women over 50. The Framingham Study. *New England Journal of Medicine* **313:** 1038–1043.

10

Treatments for menopausal and post-menopausal problems: present and future

MALCOLM WHITEHEAD

When I was asked to write this chapter the title was 'Hormone replacement therapy: present and future'. However, for reasons to be discussed, I believe that the major advances in developing effective and well tolerated treatments (associated with a high level of compliance) for menopausal and post-menopausal symptoms and diseases over the next decade will *not* be in the area of conventional oestrogen/progestogen hormone replacement therapy (HRT). Therefore, I have retitled this chapter 'Treatments for menopause and post-menopausal problems: present and future'. This chapter is divided into three sections. The first deals with some of the current 'unknowns' with HRT. These include potential beneficial effects and also some of the side effects and risks of HRT not covered elsewhere in this book. For this purpose, a side effect has been defined as an adverse effect arising, de novo, in a previously apparently healthy post-menopausal woman who has started HRT. A risk is defined as an adverse event arising in a patient with a relevant personal or family history, for example 'at risk' if HRT is prescribed. The second section deals with potential new developments in conventional oestrogen/progestogen HRT, and the third section discusses developments in non-HRT preparations for long-term use in post-menopausal women.

CURRENT 'UNKNOWNS' WITH HORMONE REPLACEMENT THERAPY

The majority of current 'unknowns' regarding hormone replacement therapy (HRT) have been covered elsewhere in this book. The more important of those that have not been discussed include:

Potential benefits of HRT

Muscle mass and strength

Muscle mass and strength decline in both men and women with advancing age; weight and the level of physical activity also influence this decline. At

Baillière's Clinical Obstetrics and Gynaecology—
Vol. 10, No. 3, September 1996
ISBN 0–7020–2177–6
0950–3552/96/030515 + 16 $12.00/00

present, it is unclear as to whether post-menopausal use of oestrogens reduces the decline in muscle strength, and contradictory data have been published (Cauley et al, 1987; Phillips et al, 1993; Preisinger et al, 1995). It is important that this issue be resolved because greater muscle mass and strength are likely to reduce not only fracture incidence but, by maintaining more vigorous exercise, may reduce the risk of cardiovascular disease (CVD).

Maintenance of collagen and prevention of skin wrinkles

It has been known for many years that oestrogen influences skin collagen content and conserves this (Brincat et al, 1985). More recently, it has been shown that oestrogen reduces collagen turnover and improves collagen quality (Holland et al, 1994). Controlled studies have shown that HRT maintains skin thickness (Maheux et al, 1994), and that topical oestrogens improve skin wrinkles (Creidi et al, 1994). The cosmetic importance of these data requires further studies as does the relationship between these findings with more medically relevant aspects of skin health, for example skin healing after surgery.

Colorectal cancer

There is increasing evidence that post-menopausal use of oestrogens reduces the risk of colorectal cancer. Both prospective cohort and case-controlled studies have reported this (Chute et al, 1991; Jacobs et al, 1994; Calle et al, 1995). A real effect is likely because the protection is greater in current compared with past users, and increases with longer durations of use. The mechanism of action is unknown.

Alzheimer's disease

Alzheimer's disease (AD) is the most frequent cause of dementia; in terms of costs it is more important than osteoporosis and CVD. Symptoms of AD can appear as early as the mid-30s but this is uncommon. Most cases occur among the elderly, with age 65 years usually being taken to demarcate early from late-onset AD. After age 65 years, the prevalence of AD increases exponentially with a doubling about every five years.

Early-onset AD is determined, to a very large extent, by genetic mutations in one of three genes: the amyloid precursor protein gene on chromosome 21, the *S182* gene on chromosome 14, and the *STM2* gene on chromosome 4 (Perick-Vance and Haines, 1995). These chromosomal abnormalities are rarely associated with late-onset disease. However, the risk of AD is strongly influenced by polymorphisms of apolipoprotein E, a plasma protein encoded by chromosome 19 and involved in lipid transport (Strittmatter et al, 1993). Despite this, and other genetic considerations, it is clear from observational studies that many factors influence the risk of AD. Evidence is growing that one exogenous factor in women is post-menopausal oestrogen deprivation.

A detailed review of the relationships between oestrogen deprivation, brain function and HRT is beyond the scope of this chapter. It suffices to say it has been suggested that HRT may not only prevent against late-onset AD, but may also improve or ameliorate the symptoms in established disease.

Evidence for the former comes from the Leisure World retirement community cohort in Southern California where prior oestrogen use was associated with a 31% lower risk of development of AD in users compared with non-users. Importantly, there were significant dose and duration effects (Paganini-Hill and Henderson, 1994). In the Baltimore Longitudinal Study of Aging, oral or transdermal use of HRT was associated with a 56% reduction in the risk of AD (Morrison et al, 1996). The results of a recent study from Seattle are more difficult to interpret; use of HRT was again associated with a lowering in risk of AD but the reduction, of 30%, was not statistically significant and no dose effect was found (Brenner et al, 1994). Clearly, further studies are urgently required to help determine the precise relationships between HRT and prevention against AD.

Currently six studies have investigated the effects of HRT in patients with established AD (Fillit et al, 1986; Honjo et al, 1989, 1993; Ohkura et al, 1994a,b,c). They must be regarded as preliminary, and none have investigated more than 15 women. Only one was a true randomized, controlled trial (Honjo et al, 1993), and only one extended treatment to beyond six weeks (Ohkura et al, 1994b). Outcome measures, for the most part, were limited to brief cognitive rating instruments. Despite these limitations, each study suggested that AD symptoms improved with oral HRT. Again, further studies which are scientifically more rigorous are urgently needed in this area.

Potential side effects of HRT

Ovarian cancer

Numerous studies on the relationships between post-menopausal oestrogen use and risk of ovarian cancer have been published. Most have investigated only small numbers of cases and therefore a pooled analysis of the literature was undertaken (Whitemore et al, 1992). This failed to show an increase in risk.

A more recent, prospective, cohort study reported no overall increase in risk with use of oestrogens. However, an increase in risk was observed when oestrogen use was continued for 11 years or more. This long-term study group comprised only 18 cases (Rodriguez et al, 1995). It is very unlikely that durations of use of HRT of 10 years or less increase the risk of ovarian cancer. More data are needed for longer durations of exposure.

Gall bladder disease

Published results are contradictory regarding gall bladder disease and HRT. The largest study which investigated the association between post-menopausal use of oestrogens and risk of gall bladder disease, the Nurses' Health Study, reported a 1.5 to 2.0 increase in risk (Grodstein et al, 1994). The risk of cholecystectomy in the Nurses' Health Study increased with both oestrogen dose and with duration of exposure. Thus, a real effect is suggested. There may also be a 'carry-over' effect after treatment is stopped which may last for up to five years.

It is not known whether non-oral routes of administration cause similar or dissimilar increases in risk. This author thinks it unlikely that non-oral oestrogens will increase risk because they do not increase bile cholesterol saturation (van Erpecum et al, 1991).

Malignant melanoma

Five studies have reported on the relationship between the use of HRT and risk of malignant melanoma (Holman et al, 1984; Osterlind et al, 1988; Adami et al, 1989; Holly et al, 1994; White et al, 1994). One case-controlled study reported a small increase in risk with long-term use of oestrogen but another case-controlled study did not (Holly et al, 1994; White et al, 1994). The other three studies reported slight increases in risk, none of which achieved statistical significance. Thus, if post-menopausal oestrogen use increases the risk then the impact is small.

It is worth noting that similar differences between small studies were found when the risk of malignant melanoma was related to the use of the combined oestrogen/progestogen contraceptive pill. The prospective cohorts of the Royal College of General Practitioners and Oxford Family Planning Association, which included adequate patient numbers and which took into account exposure to sunlight, subsequently showed no association between use of the contraceptive pill and risk of malignant melanoma (Green, 1991; Hannaford et al, 1991).

Potential risks

Fibroids and endometriosis

A detailed discussion of the relationships between oestrogens and progestogens and fibroids, and these sex hormones and endometriosis is not within the scope of this chapter. Because both fibroids and endometriotic tissue can retain sensitivity to oestrogen and progestogen, it is prudent to be mindful of the effects of HRT on these conditions.

No prospective, randomized, large-scale studies have been performed on the effects of HRT on either fibroids or endometriosis. Thus, the risk of prolonging/reactivating disease likely to be associated with significant morbidity is not known. The number and size of uterine fibroids can increase with HRT (Frigo et al, 1995). Numerous case reports link the use of HRT with the development of ovarian endometrioma, colon obstruction and obstructive uropathy. However, the latter can arise in post-menopausal women not exposed to oestrogens (Kempers et al, 1960). The only large study to investigate whether HRT increases the risk of reactivating pelvic endometriosis reported that only one of 85 women undergoing total abdominal hysterectomy and bilateral salpingo-oophorectomy, and then receiving oestradiol and testosterone implants, required further laparotomy within the first five years of treatment (Henderson and Studd, 1991).

Practical guidelines as to the management of patients with fibroids and endometriosis who receive HRT are based largely on a 'common sense' approach. Fibroid size can be monitored clinically, and the numbers can be determined by ultrasound. It would seem prudent to advise women known to have small fibroids, who are about to start HRT, to return for further examination if symptoms occur which may arise from enlarging fibroids (urinary frequency, lower abdominal or pelvic pain, increasingly heavy vaginal bleeding). Identical comments can be applied to the monitoring of patients with mild endometriosis although the type of symptom will be different (deep dyspareunia). More severe endometriotic disease may require surgery before HRT is prescribed. Current thinking is that HRT is not contraindicated in young women who have had to undergo total abdominal hysterectomy and bilateral salpingo-oophorectomy because of severe endometriosis. It is not clear whether treatment in this group of women should be oestrogen alone or oestrogen and progestogen. Testosterone can be added to either treatment, as indicated.

NEW DEVELOPMENTS IN OESTROGEN AND OESTROGEN/PROGESTOGEN HRT

Oestrogens

The past 10 to 15 years have seen very considerable developments in delivery systems for the oestrogen component of HRT. These have included transdermal delivery of oestradiol initially from a membrane-based system and more recently from a matrix dispersal system; percutaneous delivery of oestradiol from a gel, and vaginal delivery of oestradiol from both a tablet and from a ring. Buccal and sublingual routes have been evaluated but, at present, commercial preparations utilizing these routes are not believed to be planned. This is most probably because of the absence of a long-acting delivery vehicle for any oestrogen with these routes. Single dose application using the buccal or sublingual route does not provide sustained elevation of plasma oestrogens. It is unlikely that post-menopausal women will spend four hours each day masticating an oestrogen-releasing chewing gum!

Thus, fewer truly innovative developments regarding oestrogens can be expected during the next five to 10 years.

Progestogens

It is anticipated that two separate types of development will occur with progestogens: the first, the introduction of less androgenic progestogens and, the second, new routes of progestogen administration.

'New' progestogens

It has been argued that the C-21 derivatives of progesterone, such as medroxyprogesterone acetate and dydrogesterone, are to be preferred to the C-19 nortestosterone derivatives, such as norethisterone and norgestrel, because they are less likely to cause metabolic derangement. Therefore, derivatives of norgestrel have been developed which are said to give the same good cycle control; it is hoped that these derivatives, norgestimate, gestodene and desogestrel, will have less of a potentially undesirable metabolic impact.

Certain evidence supports the argument about potential differences between C-21 and C-19 derivatives but other research data do not. For example, in one epidemiological investigation the addition of a relatively high dose of oral norgestrel, 500 µg/day, sequentially to an oral oestrogen did not negate oestrogen benefits for the risk of coronary artery disease in women under 60 years of age (Falkeborn et al, 1992). At present, there are no epidemiological data which show that, when added to an oestrogen, C-21 derivatives are associated with a lower risk of CVD compared with the C-19 derivatives. The required studies have not been performed. Thus, the rationale for recommending either a C-21 derivative or one of the new generation of less androgenic C-19 derivatives comes from laboratory-based investigations in which lipid, lipoprotein, carbohydrate, thrombophilia and coagulation changes are used as surrogates for clinical disease risk.

In general, the C-21 derivatives such as medroxyprogesterone acetate, do not oppose the rise in high density lipoprotein cholesterol (HDL-C) (and particularly the HDL2 subfraction) seen with oral oestrogens (Writing Group for the PEPI Trial, 1995). The C-19 derivatives negate this rise whether given orally or transdermally (Whitcroft et al, 1994). Conversely, the C-21 derivatives do not oppose the oral oestrogen induced rise in plasma triglyceride (Writing Group for the PEPI Trial, 1995), whereas the C-19 progestogens lower triglycerides (Whitcroft et al, 1994). In the USA, it is widely believed that the 20 to 25% of arterial disease protection attributed to lipid changes with HRT is due to a rise in HDL-C and its sub-fractions. In Europe, it is believed that the lowering of triglyceride may be equally important and epidemiological data are available which show triglyceride values to be an independent risk marker for coronary heart disease (CHD) in women (Bengtsson et al, 1993). Thus, the justification for introducing less androgenic C-19 derivatives from the viewpoint of lipid and lipoprotein impact can be debated.

Data on the effects of sex hormones on carbohydrate metabolism are much sparser. However, sequential oral norgestrel has been shown to increase insulin resistance and to decrease insulin sensitivity (Godsland et al, 1993). Importantly, a C-21 derivative, medroxyprogesterone acetate, has been reported to increase insulin resistance significantly (Lindheim et al, 1993). Therefore, great care should be exercised in selecting a progestogen for adding to the oestrogen in women with impaired carbohydrate tolerance.

The new derivatives of norgestrel, which are claimed to be less androgenic are, as stated, norgestimate, gestodene and desogestrel. When added to ethinyl oestradiol in oral contraceptive formulations, these progestogens cause minimal, if any, potentially adverse metabolic impact. However, natural oestrogens, as used in HRT, are less potent than synthetic ethinyl oestradiol which is used in the combined, oral contraceptive pill. When desogestrel was added continuously (every day) to oral oestradiol in a continuous/combined HRT preparation, potentially undesirable androgenic changes in lipid and lipoprotein metabolism were observed (Marsh et al, 1994). Many metabolic advantages are anticipated with the introduction of the newer, less androgenic progestogens: whether these benefits will actually be realized remains to be seen.

Routes of administration

There can be no doubt that one of the major problems with combined, oestrogen/progestogen HRT (whether the progestogen is administered sequentially or continuously) is progestogen-induced 'pre-menstrual tension' (PMT). Because this problem appears dose-related, strategies which are aimed at reducing the daily dose appear logical.

One such approach is to avoid oral administration and to develop a system whereby the progestogen is administered non-orally but systemically. This has already been achieved with transdermal norethisterone using a membrane-based patch (Estragest: Ciba-Geigy, Basle, Switzerland). It can be confidently predicted that transdermal delivery of norethisterone and also, perhaps, norgestrel, will become available from matrix dispersal systems which, it is claimed, cause less skin irritation and adhere better than the original membrane-based patch systems.

The second approach, which also avoids oral administration, is the development of a system which releases the progestogen either within or adjacent to the endometrium and uterine cavity. Leiras has developed a norgestrel-releasing intrauterine contraceptive device (IUCD). This has already been approved for use in the UK as a contraceptive and is marketed as Mirena. It is now being evaluated for use as the progestogen component of combined oestrogen/progestogen HRT. Regrettably, norgestrel has a low 'first-pass' hepatic clearance and, therefore, although the risk of progestogen-induced physical and psychological side effects is likely to be reduced because of the low daily dose (plasma norgestrel values are approximately 200 pg/ml), lipid, lipoprotein and metabolic changes may still occur. When combined with transdermal oestradiol 50 µg/day, the norgestrel-releasing IUCD was associated with a decrease in HDL-C of 12.5% and in HDL2 cholesterol of 27% at one year (Laatikainen and Raudaskoski, 1995).

An alternative strategy has been to develop a sustained release preparation containing natural progesterone which is delivered into the upper part of the vagina. This is now registered as Crinone (Columbia Laboratories, USA). The progesterone is dissolved into a bioadhesive gel which adheres to the vaginal skin and which is inserted every 48 hours. Data presented (but not published) show that when 90 mg of progesterone is inserted every other day (six insertions over 12 days), sequentially, in combination with oral conjugated equine oestrogens (Premarin: Wyeth-Ayerst, Philadelphia, USA), uniform secretory transformation is achieved within the endometrium (Ross et al, 1996). The plasma progesterone levels are variable; some are well within the luteal phase range (approximately 30 nmol/l) but others are not (less than 10 nmol/l), yet all endometrial tissue showed evidence of good progestational activity. These data with low plasma progesterone levels suggest the existence of a 'pelvic sink'. Whether this is mediated via the lymphatic system is not known but, clearly, effective doses of progesterone are being delivered to the endometrium yet, because of the low plasma values, the risk of PMT is likely to be minimized.

Continuous/combined regimens

It has been argued that the re-establishment of vaginal bleeding with sequential therapies is one of the major reasons why women discontinue HRT. This potential problem, of course, will not be overcome using lower daily doses of progesterone/progestogen given sequentially.

The desire for amenorrhoea led to the development of continuous/combined regimens, in which the oestrogen and progestogen are both given continuously, every day. Our early experience with continuous/combined regimens incorporating conjugated equine oestrogens 0.625 mg/day and either medroxyprogesterone acetate (Provera: Upjohn, Kalamazoo, USA) 2.5 mg twice daily or norethisterone acetate (Micronor: Ortho-Cilag, High Wycombe, UK) 0.35 mg twice daily, was disappointing; approximately 50% of patients discontinued treatment either because of chronic bleeding or 'permanent PMT' (due to the continuous progestogen) by 18 months of treatment (Hillard et al, 1992). Subsequent studies of many hundreds of women by other authors have reported similarly with approximately 50% of patients having discontinued treatment at 12 months either because of chronic irregular bleeding and/or permanent PMT (Archer et al, 1994). The global experience of continuous/combined regimens has recently been critically reviewed (Udoff et al, 1995).

Whilst continuous/combined regimens may extend the use of HRT, I believe any treatment which has only a 50% compliance at 12 months could be improved upon. Hence, the hunt for 'Panaceadiol', or the development of non-HRT regimens for long-term use in post-menopausal women which will reduce the risk of osteoporotic fractures and CVD without causing endometrial proliferation and vaginal bleeding. Suppression of breast activity which might translate into a reduction in risk of breast cancer would be a bonus.

DEVELOPMENT OF NON-HRT PREPARATIONS

Two groups of non-HRT agents are currently being actively researched; the Selective Estrogen Receptor Modulators (SERMs) and phytoestrogens/soya bean extract.

SERMs

SERMs were previously called 'anti-oestrogens' and include tamoxifen (Zeneca Pharma: Wilmslow, Cheshire, UK), draloxifene (Pfizer: Sandwich, Kent, UK) and raloxifene (Eli Lilly: Indianapolis, USA). Some classifications also include certain agents which have been developed by Imperial Chemical Industries (ICI: Wilmslow, Cheshire, UK) and which are known only by number, for example ICI 182, 780 and ICI 164, 384. The latter are potent anti-oestrogens with little, if any, oestrogen agonist activity (see below). Because of this they will not be considered further here.

Tamoxifen

The principal reason for changing from 'anti-oestrogen' to 'SERM' is that the former term is inappropriate. The most well recognized action of tamoxifen is in the treatment of breast cancer. The definitive meta-analysis published in 1992 demonstrated modest but significant benefits associated with its use as an adjuvant therapy in stage 1 and stage 2 disease (Early Breast Cancer Trialists' Collaborative Group, 1992). Although the majority of women in this meta-analysis had taken tamoxifen for two years or less there was a significant trend towards greater delay of recurrence with longer-term use. Furthermore, significant benefits were seen in patients with both oestrogen receptor (ER)-positive and ER-negative tumours, although the benefits were greater in the ER-positive group.

Mode of action of tamoxifen

In very simplistic terms, tamoxifen competitively blocks oestrogen binding at the ER. The tamoxifen–ER complex will also bind to DNA, but transcription is prevented. Thus, tamoxifen is a partial agonist and, as will be seen, exhibits oestrogenic activity in certain tissues.

The observation that some women with ER-negative tumours benefit from adjuvant tamoxifen led to a more thorough investigation of its actions. In a carefully designed series of in vitro experiments, it was shown that tamoxifen increases the secretion of transforming growth factor-beta (TGF-beta) in oestrogen-responsive breast cancer cell lines (Knabbe et al, 1987). TGF-beta can inhibit the growth of ER-negative breast cancer cells. It was later shown that conventional tamoxifen therapy induces TGF-beta secretion by stromal cells from both ER-positive and ER-negative tumours in vivo, confirming that this is a truly ER-independent process (Butta et al, 1992).

Other actions of tamoxifen

Tamoxifen exerts conventional oestrogenic effects on bone mineral density and a controlled study has demonstrated spinal bone conservation in post-menopausal women with breast cancer (Love et al, 1992). Additionally, tamoxifen has also been shown to reduce the risk of death from fatal myocardial infarction. The Scottish adjuvant trial was established to determine the effects on breast cancer survival but beneficial arterial actions were also observed (McDonald and Stewart, 1991). A non-significant reduction in cardiac mortality was also observed in the Stockholm study (Rutqvist and Mattsson, 1993).

These bone and arterial effects clearly indicate oestrogenic activity. Hence the term SERM is more appropriate than anti-oestrogen. Other oestrogenic actions of tamoxifen include a stimulatory effect upon the endometrium.

The first of the large randomized studies of adjuvant tamoxifen to report on the risk of endometrial cancer was from Stockholm. This study showed a relative risk of endometrial cancer of 6.4 (95% CI 1.4–28, $P < 0.01$) in the treated patients who received tamoxifen 40 mg/day (Fornander et al, 1989). Numerous additional papers of interest in this field have been published during the past three years. Additionally, prospective studies monitoring endometrial change from the commencement of therapy, using ultrasound and histology, have confirmed that tamoxifen induces endometrial disease in up to 40% of patients (Kedar et al, 1994).

In my opinion, this uterotrophic effect of tamoxifen excludes this agent from widespread use amongst primary care physicians for prevention/treatment of osteoporosis and CVD in post-menopausal women. What, though, of the related compounds draloxifene and raloxifene?

Draloxifene and raloxifene

At this time, there are two publications relating to draloxifene and the human breast. There are no publications on other therapeutic targets, such as bone and arterial status. In a controlled, dose-finding phase II trial, draloxifene was shown to be active against advanced breast cancer (Bruning, 1992). The other study was more concerned with its pharmacokinetics and metabolism (Grill and Pollow, 1991).

More data are available on raloxifene. Much of this has been derived from in vitro and animal studies which have shown that raloxifene inhibits oestrogen stimulated MCF-7 breast cancer cell proliferation in vitro. Indeed, raloxifene is more potent than tamoxifen in this system. In mammary carcinoma cell lines which are not oestrogen dependent (the androgen sensitive Shionogi mouse mammary carcinoma model), raloxifene has no anti-proliferative activity (Thompson et al, 1988).

It has now been demonstrated that raloxifene possesses bone conserving activity. In 75-day-old ovariectomized rats, given either raloxifene or an orally available form of oestrogen daily for five weeks, it was clearly shown by both ex vivo single photon analysis of the trabecular rich region of the proximal femur, and ex vivo dual energy X-ray absorptiometry of the proximal tibial metaphysis, that raloxifene exerted a significant protective effect on bone which was statistically indistinguishable from an equivalent dose of oestrogen (Black et al, 1994). Other studies using different skeletal sites have reported similar beneficial bone effects with raloxifene (Bryant et al, 1995; Sato et al, 1995).

Raloxifene has also been shown to lower serum cholesterol (Black et al, 1994), and this effect can be maintained for at least 12 months in ovariectomized rats (Bryant et al, 1995).

Preliminary human data are now becoming available. In a double-blind, placebo-controlled, phase II clinical trial conducted in post-menopausal women, raloxifene given for two months lowered serum and urinary biochemical markers of bone metabolism in a manner similar to conjugated oestrogens at a daily dose of 0.625 mg. In this study, raloxifene also lowered total serum cholesterol and this effect was due primarily to a reduction in low density lipoprotein cholesterol (LDL-C) (Draper et al, 1993). Raloxifene did not stimulate endometrial proliferation. However, this study only lasted for two months and much longer-term data are required before it can be concluded with confidence that raloxifene will not cause endometrial disease.

Phytoestrogens

Background

Phytoestrogens are compounds derived from plants which have an affinity for the oestradiol receptor which is only five hundredth to one thousandth of that of oestradiol (Shutt and Cox, 1972; Verdeal et al, 1980). In animal models and in in vitro experimental systems, phytoestrogens, like tamoxifen and other SERMs, compete with oestradiol for the oestrogen receptor (Messina et al, 1994) and appear capable of acting as both oestrogen agonists and antagonists.

The two classes of phytoestrogens which have received most attention in relation to human health are the lignans and the isoflavones. Lignans are present in measurable levels in many fibre-rich foods while the isoflavones are confined to legumes, particularly soyabeans. Although only possessing a weak affinity for the oestradiol receptor, relatively high levels of phytoestrogens are present in food. For example, an average portion of a soya protein meal provides approximately 45 mg of isoflavones. When this is ingested each day, the urinary levels of isoflavones rise approximately 1000-fold, to up to 8000 mg/day.

Compared with caucasians in Western-style societies, Japanese women have a lower risk of CHD, breast cancer and endometrial cancer. It is tempting to speculate that these lower risks are due, at least in part, to dietary differences. Typical plasma isoflavone values of around 100 ng/ml are found in Japanese subjects who consume, on average, 50 to 100 mg of isoflavones per day from soya products. The average plasma oestradiol values of post-menopausal women in Western societies are in the range 15 to 30 pg/ml (Judd, 1976; Laufer et al, 1983). Thus, phytoestrogen levels may exceed those of endogenous oestradiol by 1000-fold.

Activity of phytoestrogens in women

In pre-menopausal women, controlled studies have shown that phyto-estrogen-rich diets (45 mg/day) modify the hormonal status and exert significant physiological effects on the regulation of the menstrual cycle (Cassidy et al, 1994, 1995). In post-menopausal women, gonadotrophin levels are reduced (Wilcox et al, 1990), and oestrogen-like changes in vaginal cytology occur (Wilcox et al, 1990) following administration of phytoestrogens.

Activity of phytoestrogens in animal models

This work has largely been carried out by the group at Bowman Gray School of Medicine, North Carolina, USA. The animal model is the cynomolgus macaque monkey fed a high cholesterol diet. Various studies have been undertaken (Anthony et al, 1996; Clarkson et al, 1996; Honore et al, 1995, 1996) which have involved feeding young macaques casein (as a control), or feeding them soy with the phytoestrogen component intact (soy+), or alternatively feeding them soy with the phytoestrogen component extracted by ethanol (soy−).

Soy+ was associated with an approximate 28% reduction in total plasma cholesterol, a 30% increase in HDL and a 30% reduction in LDL and very low density lipoprotein-cholesterol. Soy+ exerted a significantly greater effect than conjugated equine oestrogens in the elevation of HDL-C. Additionally, soy+ decreased iliac artery atherosclerosis by about 80% compared with soy− and casein. Finally, unlike conjugated equine oestrogens, soy+ enhanced the dilator responses of atherosclerotic coronary arteries to acetylcholine.

No increase in uterine weight was observed during treatment with soy+.

SUMMARY

Probable developments in HRT and non-HRT treatments for menopausal and post-menopausal problems have been reviewed.

More information is required on potential benefits and side-effects of HRT. The major potential benefit is prevention against stroke amelioration of Alzheimer's disease: the major potential side-effect discussed in this chapter is ovarian cancer.

At present, techniques for delivering oestrogens are more varied and advanced than those for progestogens. Non-oral delivery systems for progestogens which minimize side-effects will be introduced during the next decade. It is not clear whether benefits expected with new progestational agents will be realized.

Preliminary data suggest that SERMs and phytoestrogens are worthy of further evaluation. Their development will provoke intense interest over the next 10 years.

REFERENCES

Adami H-O, Persson I, Hoover R et al (1989) Risk of cancer in women receiving hormone replacement therapy. *International Journal of Cancer* **44:** 833–839.

Anthony MS, Clarkson TB, Hughes CL Jr et al (1996) Soybean isoflavones improve cardiovascular risk factors without affecting the reproductive system of peripubertal rhesus monkeys. *Journal of Nutrition* **126:** 43–50.

Archer DF, Pickar JH & Bottiglioni F (1994) Bleeding patterns in postmenopausal women taking continuous combined or sequential regimens of conjugated estrogens with medroxyprogesterone acetate. *Obstetrics and Gynecology* **83:** 686–692.

Bengtsson C, Bjorkelund C, Lapidus L & Lissner L (1993) Associations of serum lipid concentrations and obesity with mortality in women: 20 year follow-up of participants in prospective population study in Gothenberg, Sweden. *British Medical Journal* **307:** 1385–1388.

Black LJ, Sato M, Rowley ER et al (1994) Raloxifene (LY139481 HCI) prevents bone loss and reduces serum cholesterol without causing uterine hypertrophy in ovariectomized rats. *Journal of Clinical Investigation* **93:** 63–69.

Brenner DE, Kukull WA, Stergachis A et al (1994) Postmenopausal estrogen replacement therapy and the risk of Alzheimer's disease: a population-based case-control study. *American Journal of Epidemiology* **140:** 262–267.

Brincat M, Moniz C, Studd JWW et al (1985) Long-term effects of the menopause and sex hormones on skin thickness. *British Journal of Obstetrics and Gynaecology* **92:** 256–259.

Bruning PF (1992) Draloxifene, a new anti-oestrogen in postmenopausal advanced breast cancer: preliminary results of a double-blind, dose-finding phase II trial. *European Journal of Cancer* **28A(8/9):** 1404–1407.

Bryant HU, Turner CH, Frolik CA et al (1995) Long term effects of raloxifene (LY139478 HCI) on bone, cholesterol and uterus in ovariectomized rats. *Bone* **16 (supplement):** 116S. (Abstract).

Butta A, MacLennan K, Flanders KC et al (1992) Induction of transforming growth factor beta-1 in human breast cancer in vivo following tamoxifen treatment. *Cancer Research* **52:** 4261–4264.

Calle EE, Miracle-McMahill HL, Thun MJ & Health CW Jr (1995) Estrogen replacement therapy and risk of fatal colon cancer in a prospective cohort of postmenopausal women. *Journal of the National Cancer Institute* **87:** 517–523.

Cassidy A, Bingham S & Setchell K (1994) Biological effects of isoflavones present in soy in premenopausal women: implications for the prevention of breast cancer. *American Journal of Clinical Nutrition* **60:** 333–340.

Cassidy A, Bingham S & Setchell K (1995) Biological effects of isoflavones in young women—importance of the chemical composition of soya products. *British Journal of Nutrition* **74:** 587–601.

Cauley JA, Petrini AM, LaPorte RE et al (1987) The decline of grip strength in the menopause: relationship to physical activity, estrogen use and anthropometric factors. *Journal of Chronic Diseases* **40:** 115–120.

Chute CG, Willett WC, Colditz GA et al (1991) A prospective study of reproductive history and exogenous estrogens on the risk of colorectal cancer in women. *Epidemiology* **2:** 201–207.

Clarkson TB, Anthony MS, Williams JK et al (in press) The potential of soybean phytoestrogens for postmenopausal hormone replacement therapy. *Proceedings of the Society for Experimental Biology and Medicine*

Creidi P, Faivre B, Agache P et al (1994) Effect of a conjugated oestrogen (Premarin) cream on ageing facial skin. A comparative study with a placebo cream. *Maturitas* **19:** 211–223.

Draper MW, Flowers DE, Huster WJ et al (1993) Effects of raloxifene (LY139481) on biochemical markers of bone and lipid metabolism in healthy postmenopausal women. In Christiansen C & Riis B (eds) Proceedings of the Fourth International Symposium on Osteoporosis and Consensus Development Conference, pp 119–121. Aalborg, Denmark: Handelstrykkeriet Aalborg Aps.

Early Breast Cancer Trialists' Collaborative Group (1992) Systemic treatment of early breast cancer by hormonal, cytotoxic or immune therapy. *Lancet* **339:** 1–15, 71–85.

Falkeborn M, Persson I, Adami H-O et al (1992) The risk of acute myocardial infarction after oestrogen and oestrogen–progestogen replacement. *British Journal of Obstetrics and Gynaecology* **99:** 821–828.

Fillit H, Weinreb H, Cholst I et al (1986) Observations in a preliminary open trial of estradiol therapy for senile dementia—Alzheimer's type. *Psychoneuroendocrinology* **11:** 337–345.

Fornander T, Rutqvist LE, Cedermark B et al (1989) Adjuvant tamoxifen in early breast cancer: occurrence of new primary cancers. *Lancet* **i**: 117–120.

Frigo P, Eppel W, Asseryanis F et al (1995) The effects of hormone substitution in depot form on the uterus in a group of 50 peri-menopausal women—a vaginosonographic study. *Maturitas* **21**: 221–225.

Godsland I, Gangar K, Walton C et al (1993) Insulin resistance, secretion and elimination in postmenopausal women receiving oral or transdermal hormone replacement therapy. *Metabolism* **42**: 846–853.

Green A (1991) Oral contraceptives and skin neoplasia. *Contraception* **43**: 653–666.

Grill HJ & Pollow K (1991) Pharmacokinetics of draloxifene and its metabolites in breast cancer patients. *American Journal of Clinical Oncology* **14 (supplement 2)**: S21–S29.

Grodstein F, Colditz GA & Stampfer MJ (1994) Postmenopausal hormone use and cholecystectomy in a large prospective study. *Obstetrics and Gynecology* **83**: 5–11.

Hannaford PC, Villard-Mackintosh L, Vessey MP & Kay CR (1991) Oral contraceptives and malignant melanoma. *British Journal of Cancer* **63**: 430–433.

Henderson AF & Studd JWW (1991) The role of definitive surgery and hormone replacement therapy in the treatment of endometriosis. In Thomas EJ & Rock JA (eds) *Modern Approaches to Endometriosis*, pp 275–290. London: Kluwer.

Hillard TC, Siddle NC, Whitehead MI et al (1992) Continuous combined conjugated equine estrogen–progestogen therapy: effects of medroxyprogesterone acetate and norethindrone acetate on bleeding patterns and endometrial histologic diagnosis. *American Journal of Obstetrics and Gynecology* **167**: 1–7.

Holland EFN, Studd JWW, Mansell JP et al (1994) Changes in collagen composition and cross-links in bone and skin of osteoporotic postmenopausal women treated with percutaneous estradiol implants. *Obstetrics and Gynecology* **83**: 180–183.

Holly EA, Cress RD & Ahn DK (1994) Cutaneous melanoma in women: ovulatory life, menopause and use of exogenous estrogens. *Cancer Epidemiology, Biomarkers, Prevention* **661**: 668.

Holman CDJ, Armstrong BK & Heenan PJ (1984) Cutaneous malignant melanoma in women: exogenous sex hormones and reproductive factors. *British Journal of Cancer* **50**: 673–680.

Honjo H, Ogino Y, Naitoh K et al (1989) In vivo effects by estrone sulfate on the central nervous system—senile dementia (Alzheimer's type). *Journal of Steroid Biochemistry* **34**: 521–525.

Honjo H, Ogino Y, Tanaka K et al (1993) An effect of conjugated estrogen to cognitive impairment in women with senile dementia—Alzheimer's type: a placebo-controlled double blind study. *Journal of the Japan Menopause Society* **1**: 167–171.

Honore EK, Williams JK & Anthony MS (1995) Enhancement of coronary vasodilation by soy phytoestrogens and genistein. *Circulation* **92 (supplement I)**: 349 (Abstract).

Honore EK, Williams JK, Anthony MS et al (in press) Dietary soybean isoflavones prevent intimal hyperplasia after arterial injury in atherosclerotic nonhuman primates. *Journal of Vascular Surgery*

Jacobs EJ, White E & Weiss NS (1994) Exogenous hormones, reproductive history, and colon cancer. *Cancer Causes Control* **5**: 359–365.

Judd HL (1976) Hormonal dynamics associated with the menopause. *Clinical Obstetrics and Gynaecology* **19**: 775.

Kedar RP, Bourne TH, Powles TJ et al (1994) Effects of tamoxifen on uterus and ovaries of postmenopausal women in a randomised breast cancer prevention trial. *Lancet* **343**: 1318–1321.

Kempers RD, Dockerty MB, Hunt AB et al (1960) Significant postmenopausal endometriosis. *Surgical Gynaecology and Obstetrics* **111**: 348–356.

Knabbe C, Lippman ME, Wakefield LM et al (1987) Evidence that transforming growth factor-beta is a hormonally regulated negative growth factor in human breast cancer cells. *Cell* **48**: 417–428.

Laatikainen T & Raudaskoski T (1995) Hormone replacement therapy with levonorgestrel-releasing intrauterine device and transdermal estrogen: Clinical, endometrial and lipid responses. Presentation at the European Consensus Meeting on Menopause, Montreux, September 1995.

Laufer LR, DeFazio JL & Lu JKH (1983) Estrogen replacement therapy by transdermal estradiol administration. *American Journal of Obstetrics and Gynecology* **146**: 533.

Lindheim SR, Presser SC, Ditkoff EC et al (1993) A possible bimodal effect of estrogen on insulin sensitivity in postmenopausal women and the attenuating effect of added progestin. *Fertility and Sterility* **60**: 664–667.

Love RR, Mazess RB, Barden HS et al (1992) Effects of tamoxifen on bone mineral density in postmenopausal women with breast cancer. *New England Journal of Medicine* **326**: 852–856.

McDonald CC & Stewart HJ (1991) Fatal myocardial infarction in the Scottish adjuvant tamoxifen trial. *British Medical Journal* **303:** 435–437.

Maheux R, Naud F, Rioux M et al (1994) A randomised, double-blind, placebo-controlled study on the effect of conjugated estrogens on skin thickness. *American Journal of Obstetrics and Gynecology* **170:** 642–649.

Marsh MS, Crook D, Whitcroft SI et al (1994) Effect of continuous combined estrogen and desogestrel hormone replacement therapy on serum lipids and lipoproteins. *Obstetrics and Gynecology* **83:** 19–23.

Messina MJ, Persky V, Setchell KDR & Barnes S (1994) Soy intake and cancer risk: a review of the in vitro and in vivo data. *Nutrition and Cancer* **21:** 113.

Morrison A, Resnick S, Corrada M et al (1996) A prospective study of estrogen replacement therapy and the risk of developing Alzheimer's disease in the Baltimore longitudinal study of aging. *Neurology* **46:** A435–A436. (Abstract).

Ohkura T, Isse K, Akazawa K et al (1994a) An open trial of estrogen therapy for dementia of the Alzheimer type in women. In Berg G & Hammar M (eds) *The Modern Management of the Menopause: A Perspective for the 21st Century*, pp 315–333. New York: Parthenon.

Ohkura T, Isse K, Akazawa K et al (1994b) Low dose estrogen replacement therapy for Alzheimer disease in women. *Menopause* **1:** 125–130.

Ohkura T, Isse K, Akazawa K et al (1994c) Evaluation of estrogen treatment in female patients with dementia of the Alzheimer type. *Endocrine Journal* **41:** 361–371.

Osterlind A, Tucker MA, Stone BJ & Jensen OM (1988) The Danish case-control study of cutaneous malignant melanoma. III. Hormonal and reproductive factors in women. *International Journal of Cancer* **42:** 821–824.

Paganini-Hill A & Henderson V (1994) Estrogen deficiency and risk of Alzheimer's disease in women. *American Journal of Epidemiology* **140:** 256–261.

Perick-Vance MA & Haines JL (1995) Genetic susceptibility to Alzheimer disease. *Trends in Genetics* **11:** 504–508.

Phillips SK, Rook KM, Siddle NC et al (1993) Muscle weakness in women occurs at an earlier age than in men, but strength is preserved by hormone replacement therapy. *Clinical Science* **84:** 95–98.

Preisinger E, Alacamlioglu Y, Saradeth T et al (1995) Forearm bone density and grip strength in women after menopause, with and without estrogen replacement therapy. *Maturitas* **21:** 57–63.

Rodriguez C, Calle EE, Coates RJ et al (1995) Estrogen replacement therapy and fatal ovarian cancer. *American Journal of Epidemiology* **141:** 828–835.

Ross D, Pryse-Davies J, Collins WP & Whitehead MI (1996) Randomised, double-blind, endometrial study of a vaginal progesterone gel in oestrogen-treated postmenopausal women. Abstract presented at the 8th International Congress on the Menopause, Sydney, Australia.

Rutqvist LE & Mattsson A (1993) Cardiac and thromboembolic morbidity among postmenopausal women with early-stage breast cancer in a randomised trial of adjuvant tamoxifen. *Journal of the National Cancer Institute* **85:** 1398–1406.

Sato M, Kim J, Short LL et al (1995) Longitudinal and cross-sectional analysis of raloxifene effects on tibiae from ovariectomized aged rats. *Journal of Pharmacological Experimental Therapy* **272:** 1252–1259.

Shutt DA & Cox RI (1972) Steroid and phytoestrogen binding to sheep uterine receptors in vitro. *Journal of Endocrinology* **52:** 299–310.

Strittmatter WJ, Saunders AM, Schmechel D et al (1993) Apolipoprotein E: high-avidity binding to B-amyloid and increased frequency of type 4 allele in late-onset familial Alzheimer disease. *Proceedings of the National Academy of Sciences of the USA* **90:** 1977–1981.

Thompson EW, Reich R, Shima TB et al (1988) Differential regulation of growth and invasiveness of MCF-7 breast cancer cells by anti-estrogens. *Cancer Research* **48:** 6764–6768.

Udoff L, Langenberg P & Adashi EY (1995) Combined continuous hormone replacement therapy: a critical review. *Obstetrics and Gynecology* **86:** 306–316.

van Erpecum KJ, van Berge Henegouwen GP, Verschoor L et al (1991) Different hepatobiliary effects of oral and transdermal estradiol in postmenopausal women. *Gastroenterology* **100:** 482–488.

Verdeal K, Brown RR, Richardson T & Ryan DS (1980) Affinity of phytoestrogens for estradiol-binding proteins and effect of coumestrol on growth of 7, 12-dimethylbenz (alpha) anthracene-induced rat mammary tumours. *Journal of the National Cancer Institute* **64:** 285–290.

Whitcroft SIJ, Crook D, Marsh MS et al (1994) Long-term effects of oral and transdermal hormone replacement therapies on serum lipid and lipoprotein concentrations. *Obstetrics and Gynecology* **84:** 222–226.

White E, Kirkpatrick CS & Lee JAH (1994) Case-control study of malignant melanoma in Washington State. 1. Constitutional factors and sun exposure. *American Journal of Epidemiology* **139:** 857–868.

Whittemore AS, Harris R, Itnyre J and the Collaborative Ovarian Cancer Group (1992) Characteristic relation to ovarian cancer risk: collaborative analysis of twelve US case-control studies. II. Invasive epithelial ovarian cancers in white women. *American Journal of Epidemiology* **136:** 1184–1203.

Wilcox G, Wahlqvist ML, Burger HG & Medley G (1990) Oestrogen effects of plant derived foods in postmenopausal women. *British Medical Journal* **301:** 905–906.

The Writing Group for the PEPI Trial (1995) Effects of estrogen and estrogen/progestin regimens on heart disease risk factors in postmenopausal women: the Postmenopausal Estrogen/Progestin Interventions (PEPI) Trial. *Journal of the American Medical Association* **273:** 199–208.

Index

Note: Page numbers of article titles are in **bold** type.